Real life experiences from
important it is to speak up anc

Edited by Jo Baldwin Trott

Being FINE

THE OTHER 'F' WORD

In support of MyBlackDog.co

PROPER BOOKS

First published January 2021 © Proper Books

Disclaimer: *Being FINE* is intended for information and education purposes only. This book does not constitute specific legal, financial, clinical or commercial advice unique to your situation.

The views and opinions expressed in this book are those of the authors and do not reflect those of the Publisher and Resellers, who accept no responsibility for loss, damage or injury to persons or their belongings as a direct or indirect result of reading this book.

All people mentioned in case studies have been used with permission, and/or have had names, genders, industries and personal details altered to protect client confidentiality. Any resemblance to persons living or dead is purely coincidental.

A CIP catalogue record for this book is available from the British Library.

Published by Proper Books

properbookspublishing@gmail.com

ISBN: 978-1-8383359-0-8

Contents

Foreword

Niki Clarke
Founder of My Black Dog Charity

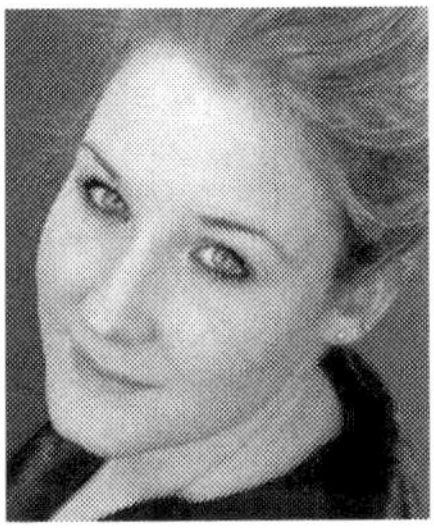

It is a pleasure to be asked to contribute to this incredible book and be a part of the many voices that have bravely spoken to share their stories.

I founded the mental health charity, My Black Dog, to help people come forward and feel safe when talking about the struggles they are having. One of the most debilitating parts of suffering with your mental health is the anguish that comes with opening up and being honest with others about what you are going through. For me, I never wanted to reach into my soul and drag out the darkness that has raged in there for so long; I thought I would be judged, or left, or pitied. I thought

I would scare people away and that they would forever see me differently. Most of all, I thought I would always be alone in my struggles, a solitary creature dealing with depression: dark, monstrous, alone.

I have, however, felt privileged to hear the many tales of mental health difficulties that are in this book. I know how hard mental health is to talk about – the fear you feel when you expose yourself, the longing you feel to be accepted, to feel happy, to feel safe. These stories are incredible; they show the raw, brutal reality of living with mental illness. So I say to each of the contributors who have been so brave in sharing their story, thank you. To the readers, I say, you are not alone. Even in the darkest of times, you are never alone.

It is only by coming together and talking about our experiences that we can shed a light on the devastating effects of mental illness. To each person who can speak up and talk openly about this, you are an inspiration for someone else to do the same. In these cases, the difference between talking and staying silent can be one of life and death.

My Black Dog is an online peer-to-peer chat function run entirely by volunteers with lived experiences. They really do understand what you are going through. When you don't know who to talk to, talk to someone who gets it.

Please get in touch with us, we are here for you.

www.myblackdog.co

Being FINE

Real life experiences from those who know how important it is to speak up and share how we really feel

Dare to be Sensitive

Kapil Gupta

There is an increasing amount of focus on men's mental health and wellbeing at the moment. Last year I was invited to deliver a Men's Connection Workshop at one of the large government organisations in London.

The first thing I noticed was the feeling of uneasiness amongst the men in the room. The group was made up of men ranging in age from mid-twenties to mid-sixties. There was an awkward sense that they had been forced to be in the workshop as part of a tick-box exercise. It felt like they didn't want to be in the room.

This is not uncommon when a group of men get together with the purpose to purely connect and not to discuss sports, politics, news, work, etc.

Men's discomfort with connection is not a new thing for me after leading Men's Groups and workshops, and coaching men one-on-one and in group scenarios, for over seven years.

Soon everyone was seated and I started explaining why I was there, my work with men and why the connection was important. I could see everyone's eyes glazing over and that nobody was interested in what I had to say. They were all pretty engrossed in their discomfort and waiting for me to sell them something.

I paused and said: 'Why don't we take some time and connect? I want to hear from you guys. Let's start by saying something about how you are feeling right now.'

And then one by one they all started saying the two most dreaded words in the history of human connection – 'I am *good*', and 'I am *fine*'.

After about ten people had said the same words, I had to ask them to stop. I said, part-joking and part-serious, 'Since when do men have just two words in our vocabulary to describe our feelings?'

You could feel the discomfort and confusion in the room.

After what seemed like ages, one guy spoke up: 'I feel like I can't say how I feel because I don't want to burden anyone with my feelings!'

Everyone else in the room silently nodded in agreement. The permission to be vulnerable had just entered the room.

Another guy spoke up: 'I feel that if I tell someone how I am feeling, it will leave me exposed and they could take advantage of me.'

And there you have it – the two most common themes I see again and again in all my men's groups and coaching with men. We are walking around trying to perform, trying to please, trying to prove to the world that we are good enough and that we are 'man' enough. All the while, we don't believe we can share how we feel with anyone because we do not want to burden anyone.

We have been programmed to see that this world is not a safe place. It is not safe to be sensitive and vulnerable. If we open up to anyone, we have to watch our backs as some monster is lurking around the corner waiting to stab us.

I believe that a guarded life is a terrible life to live.

One of my teachers used to ask everyone this question in his men's workshops: 'Are you a good man?' It was rare for anyone to answer that question with a straight 'Yes'. It isn't because these were bad men. It is because when you ask a man that question he searches his brain for all the places where he hasn't been good enough, where he could have done a better job, or where he didn't meet his own and society's standards of what a 'good' man should be!

We live in a culture where as men we feel we need to prove our self-worth, our value ... before we can admit that we are good men. We carry this invisible burden to protect people from our feelings because we do not want to add to their existing pain. We silently carry the burden of trying to be good enough to provide and protect our loved ones because that is what our society conditions us to do.

This is not to say that it is only men who face these issues. However, I do believe – and this is also my personal experience – that generally speaking it is men who are conditioned this way.

The education around our inherent goodness, our inherent self-worth and value is missing from our education. Very early on in our lives, we are taught to compete and derive our self-worth, our inner value by being better than others, by achieving things, by succeeding in life.

If I don't succeed, if I am not better than …, if I am not top of the class or top of the race then I am a loser.

It's not that these traits are not important; success and achievement are important parts of living in the modern world. However, what should be one half of the equation becomes the entire formula, and we end up losing our identity in the rat race and then behaving like robots.

I have lived most of my life like that.

I was a very sensitive child. I remember times when I would cry as a young boy and my parents would tell me that if I cried other kids would make fun of me.

One summer, while growing up in India, my cousins came to stay at our house during the summer vacation. I was probably seven or eight years old then. When they were leaving, I felt really sad and couldn't bring myself to go see them off. My mother saw me sitting by myself, feeling sad and crying. She came up to me and said, 'How are you going to live in this world if you are this sensitive?'

At that moment I created a belief that being that sensitive was somehow wrong. My mother wanted to protect me. She had no idea what impact it would have on me, but I distinctly remember thinking to myself at that moment, 'I will never let myself feel this way ever again.'

I believe I created a safety shield in front of my heart that day.

From then on anytime my heart would get broken or I went through intense negative emotions, I would say to myself, 'I will never let myself feel this way ever again.'

Every time I would go through a similar experience, I would build up yet another layer of fortification on top of my heart.

I was very successful in the end. After a while, nothing could touch me. I became the ideal stoic man. I never allowed myself to feel any sadness or anger or any so-called negative emotions. I was 'cool as a cucumber' and very proud of it.

What I didn't realise though is that along the way I had forgotten who I was. I was living a life based on how other people wanted me to be – a life of how I 'should' be.

The first time I got an inclination that something was probably wrong was when my father passed away as a result of an accident in 2002. I was 25. I couldn't bring myself to cry after his death. I had responsibilities so got even more into living a functional life. At the back of my mind, I felt that something was missing but I couldn't say what it was. I did not have much time to pay attention to what was happening at the time.

It took another ten years and the loss of my first marriage to get to a level of desperation where I realised something wasn't right.

I was living life in a narrow bandwidth of emotions, never allowing myself to feel any emotional pain and, on the other side, not feeling any joy or happiness either. I was scared that if I allowed myself to feel joy, then something would go wrong and I would end up feeling a lot of pain again, and that was something to be avoided at all costs by staying guarded and alert. I didn't realise at the time but it was emotionally exhausting to hold so much in.

I had to do something to change. It dawned on me that I had to take immediate action, that if I didn't do something about it at that moment, then another five or ten years down the line, I would be living a numbed-out life and would likely have gone through yet more cycles of achievement and another relationship. And all the while I was wondering if there were more to life than the experience I was having – a life that had no mystery, a hollow life, a life that looked good on paper but had all the joy sucked out of it.

The question that I had to ask myself was, 'If not now then when?'

That decision led me to a new path, a deep dive into self-awareness, a deep dive into my belief system and how I came to create my identity. I started to see how I had grown up learning the tools to live in the adult world without ever really learning the emotional maturity that was required to go with it. I had accumulated a war chest of skills to impress people and get ahead in the commercial world, but I was still a boy when it came to my emotions and connections with people.

We are never taught that connection is an absolute necessity in every part of our lives – be that family, friends, relationships, working with colleagues or our clients, or meeting people in social environments.

That journey helped me to see how I had designed my life so that people could look at me from the outside and say, 'He has made it in life'. I had checked all the boxes so that my friends and family would feel happy about my achievements. Anytime I met a stranger, I could list my achievements to impress them. I had done a great job of acquiring things – career, money, material things, relationship, marriage. Yet, I had no clue how to be in a relationship with any of them.

Early on in my journey, someone asked me a very simple question: 'What do you want in life?' I couldn't find an answer. I knew what I didn't want, but I had no idea what I wanted. Underneath all of that, I realised that I had no idea who I was.

As I learned more about myself, I started to see all the places I had put up a shield in front of my heart to protect myself. I started to see that when I was honest, authentic and vulnerable with people I was able to develop deeper, more intimate connections. I started to learn about my boundaries. I started to take risks and open myself up with people so that they could feel the real me underneath all the safety and defence mechanisms. I surrounded myself with like-minded people who wanted the same.

I had to unlearn all the ways my ego had built the safety mechanisms around my heart to keep me safe and guarded.

Over time, I started to see that my vulnerability was only a weakness if I believed what society was telling me. My experience of vulnerability became one of strength and not weakness. I learned that I did not need to be right when I was arguing. As soon as I gave up the need to be right, the connection with people around me deepened.

I learned that heartbreak was part of life and one of the places where we feel most alive.

So, when I saw these men in the workshop starting to get vulnerable, I gave them a prompt. I asked them to think of a time when they were young, and they got hurt and closed their heart – a time when they decided to protect themselves and not allow themselves to feel that way again. I told them the story of my father passing and how I wasn't able to feel anything. I asked them what they would do differently if they were to allow their heart to be open.

It was as if a light switch got flipped at that moment in the room. One of the guys in the room said, 'I have a best friend, but I have never really told him that he is my best friend. I have never even thought about it until now and I am going to tell him that when I next see him.'

Another guy said, pointing to one of his colleagues in the room, 'He is my best friend and I have never told him that and how much his friendship means to me.'

It was as if we opened the tap that had been turned off for a long time. Slowly everyone in the room started to open up and connect. You could feel the warm, thick electricity in the room that is present when people feel connected and emotionally intimate with each other. There was a sense of brotherhood in that room. I was reminded of how easy it is to find a connection if we are willing to let our guards down and open our hearts to each other.

I also see this happening when any new men join the men's groups that I facilitate. Men's groups have an atmosphere that is rooted in vulnerability, openness, sensitivity and accountability. New people are shocked, surprised and awed at how easy it is for them to open up and share their feelings, quite often even when they haven't done so for a long time.

I often get asked this question by men: 'It is really easy to open up in Men's Groups in the company of like-minded men. How do I have these kinds of conversations with my friends?' Therein lies the sensitivity and desire for connection and the tenderness that goes with, 'I want to experience emotional intimacy with my friends, and I feel unskilled at it. Please help!'

I feel that each one of us has to take responsibility for healing our hearts. We have to stop using our past experiences as an excuse to not take this responsibility. We have to then show up to hold space for other men. All it takes is one act of courage to show up vulnerably and with an open heart and then you build from there.

I feel that this is paramount in today's culture – a culture where men are continuously bombarded with marketing messages about how to fit into a box to be 'man enough'. We need to create opportunities where men can be in approval of their emotions and feelings amongst other men, where they are not shamed or made to feel 'less than' for their vulnerability and sensitivity. If we don't do that then we will continue to see men who are numbed out and stressed out, men who are continuously chasing the next shiny object to prove their self-worth and their manliness, all the while going deeper and deeper into the downward spiral of stress and mental health issues.

This is a call to men – dare to be sensitive!

About Kapil

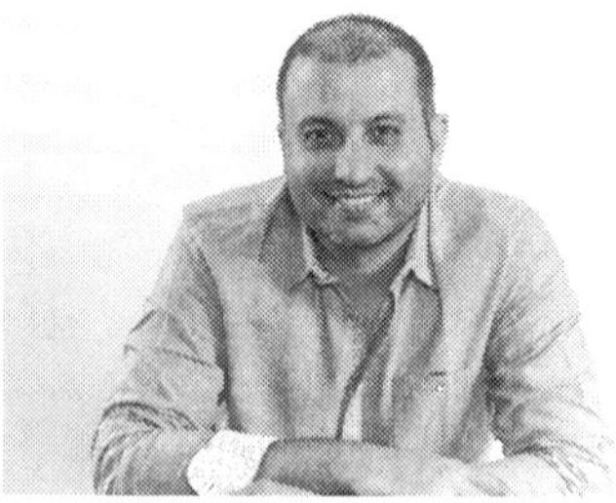

Founder of Nibana.life, Kapil Gupta is a Master Coach and a TEDx Speaker. He helps successful entrepreneurs and business executives to find joy, purpose, intimacy, satisfying relationships and fulfilment in life.

Kapil went through major personal transformation after a successful corporate career of more than 15 years, an MBA from the University of Edinburgh, and a failed marriage.

Committing himself to mastery of a new paradigm of relationships, which included how to be authentic, vulnerable, and in approval of the so-called negative aspects of his personality, Kapil's journey of personal growth took him away from corporate life and transformed him into a transformation and men's interpersonal skills coach.

Kapil co-founded TurnON Britain, a company dedicated towards personal growth, for which he also raised $1m in capital. He spent six years living a very spiritually monastic lifestyle, full of practices based in connection and relating.

He has taught more than a thousand people in workshops and coached more than a hundred.

Connect with Kapil

www.linkedin.com/in/kapilgupta (personal)

www.linkedin.com/company/nibana-life (Nibana)

www.instagram.com/kapsgupta/?hl=en (personal)

www.instagram.com/nibana.life/?hl=en (Nibana)

www.facebook.com/kapsgupta (personal)

www.facebook.com/nibana.life (Nibana)

www.nibana.life/

www.twitter.com/Kapsg

A Mountain Climbed

Simon Walker

When I was invited to write for this book it could not have come at a more opportune time. Rather inconvenient, but opportune nevertheless. I will explain more about that later.

My journey has been a long one – not an overnight success but a long meandering one of steady growth, learning and opening up. Sometimes I was moving forward but as often as not I was taking a side step or even a back step, if I was not ready for the life lesson that was coming.

So, let's start 13 years ago. At that point I had been married for 18 years with two fabulous sons. I was a town councillor, had my own shop-fitting business, and a four bedroom house. I was 'tight head prop forward' for the local town's rugby club and had a plentiful social life. Then, as happens with many marriages, we got divorced and I moved away.

I was now standing in an empty flat in a strange town where I did not know a soul. I had been divorced for two years; my then partner had just left me with the words, 'You are just too nice.' I went from being a man that seemingly had everything to a man standing in an empty flat with nothing. Going from happy to painfully sad had seemed to take a nanosecond. I was worthless, or that is how I felt at the time.

My depression came from nowhere. I had never experienced anything like it before and it slowly and insidiously wrapped around me like a python. It tightened around my chest and stopped my normal breath. I felt as though it had been replaced with a little flutter of breath, barely delivering enough oxygen to stay conscious. The flat I was standing in became my nemesis. It was a mirror of me: cold, empty and silent. So very silent. Night after night of nothingness, truly little sleep, just listening to every negative thought shouting in my ear: worthless, stupid, fat, idiot, poor, terrible son/brother. Night after night, it was the same thing.

I was still working, though not for myself anymore. I worked for a building company who were renovating an old office block into flats. It was a busy site full of tradesmen, but I had never felt so lonely. No one knew what I was going through, and they were not interested. 'Cor! Bloody hell, you look terrible!' And I would reply: 'Nar, I'm fine.' Considering the name of this book it sounds like a cliché but that was the standard conversation. I would frequently find a quiet room, wedge the door shut, curl up in the foetal position and long for sleep to come. Then at the end of the day I'd return home to an empty cold flat.

It was not long before the darkest of dark thoughts would come. Let's face it, I had nothing to offer the world. It would be better not to be here. I considered in detail (as I am rather a practical man) how to exit stage left. Overdose? Jumping? Nope, this would not do. Can you imagine how it would be for the boys growing up knowing their father committed suicide?

Make it look like an accident, I thought. Mess up the flat, make it look like a break-in and run onto a knife. Oh God, no! Far too painful!

That Friday, a typical autumnal day, I finished work early, drove home and like many other evenings I did not turn into the cul-de-sac where I lived. I knew the dread I would feel stepping into the flat so I would sometimes drive for miles before returning. Today was different. I kept driving. I drove all the way to Snowdonia to a lovely place called Betws-y-coed, and I booked into a wonderful B&B. The next morning I came downstairs, had breakfast, gathered my things, and filled in the mountain register with my estimated time of return. I started my assent on the Watkins track with no intention of returning that day. My teenage boys would be blissfully unaware their father had committed suicide. Instead, the slightly stubborn man went for a walk up a mountain, got lost and succumbed to hypothermia. After all, that was far less painful than a knife. Apparently dying of hypothermia was not that bad at all. I was finally going to get a good night's sleep and silence the negative voices in my head.

Nearing the top was treacherous that day. It sounds silly but I was scared as the weather was so bad. I was floundering around in knee-deep snow when out of the bleakness a man dressed in full mountain gear turned up. Seeing I was in trouble and badly prepared for the conditions he suggested we buddied up and walked down the mountain to safety. He will never know what he did for me that day. However, that was the wakeup call I needed. As Joseph Campbell states in the Hero's Journey, it was my call to adventure. It was like a slap around the face with a freezing cold North Atlantic cod.

Scared and alone back in my flat I rang the local doctors and made an appointment. I remember to this day walking into Dr Silver's room. I'm a big strapping man but to Dr Silver I must have looked like a scared lost puppy. 'So, Mr Walker, it looks like we need to talk,' he said, and I burst into tears. And there I was for well over my five minutes. With love, empathy and compassion he sat and listened to a blubbering snotty mess of a man. This was the first time I had ever shared how I truly felt, and it felt like the Universe had been lifted off my shoulders. Once he had referred me to a psychotherapist he let me out of the side door to save my embarrassment of being seen by the waiting patients. I stepped out into dappled sunlight shining through the autumn trees. That moment felt magical, as if I could have walked on the clouds.

Someone just listening to me for 20 minutes had changed my life. Thank you, Dr Silver, from the bottom of my heart.

Who would have thought that we, as the human species, would have evolved to have such a negative bias? I, for one, did not. Without it, though, we would have been really rubbish at surviving. We would have thought the dark shadow behind the rose bush was a cute kitten, and then would have been eaten by the sabre-toothed tiger that stepped out. This negativity bias and the fight-and-flight response served us jolly well for thousands of years. However, modern life does not have so many near-death experiences any more when we pop out to the shops to hunt and gather. Instead the hippocampus and amygdala parts of our brain work like the clappers, making stuff up, giving us false information until we give ourselves a DIY frontal lobotomy.

Our brains basically play with us just because they are bored. Of course, I am making light of this fantastic part of human evolution and it is far more scientific and hugely more interesting and involved than I have explained. However, after a few sessions with a psychotherapist who really knew about this stuff, I realised what I had gone through was just part of the human condition. It was not my weakness, it was not shameful, it was just being human. Everyone goes through it, every single day. We just need to get to know those thoughts and know they are not real. They are based on the past and are imaginings of the future. We absolutely need to know it's OK to feel shitty and we absolutely need to talk to people about it. Especially us men. It does not matter how big we are, how 'hard' we are, we are all human and we are all wired the same way.

In the last few months before receiving therapy, I had not been open to any of the positives that had happened. I had let my negativity rule the roost. I had not remembered the neighbour who had come over to give me a microwave hours after I had moved into my empty flat. He had said: 'Hope you don't mind but I saw you move in and thought you might like this to get you started again.' He had been in my shoes a few years earlier.

My brother would also phone me in the middle of the night, knowing I was not sleeping, and would read me poetry. Again he had been in the same place that I was in. These are just a few of many beautiful acts of kindness I had not noticed in the depths of my depression.

I lived in that flat for a further six months and loved every minute. The flat had not changed, just my way of thinking. I left the radio on when I went out and I bought a slow cooker so I came home to the smell of fresh cooking and Radio 4. What more could a man want? Now, I am not saying it was all sweetness and light; far from it. Life can still get really shitty at times. I saved like mad to put a deposit down on a new life in North Devon, an adorable place, and close to a couple of dear friends who had reached out to me and lent me their pink sparkly bits. (Just ask me anytime and I will be more than happy to tell you about pink sparkly bits. I may even lend you some of mine.)

I moved again in 2008, just before the banks crashed. Long story short, I gave the property back to the bank. They obviously needed it more than I did! Then I walked headlong into what I know now was a co-dependent relationship with a narcissist, so I lost my confidence for a while.

My car was stolen along with £4000 worth of tools, and then I stood by my mother's hospital bed as she drew her final breath. This was one of the most beautiful things I have ever experienced, but again I will have to tell you about this another time. Never did I slip into the spiral of despair again. I had built a coping mechanism, an emotional intelligence and a flexibility that was serving me, not enslaving me. I was getting there one step at a time.

I had learnt not to outsource my happiness or unhappiness on external things but to accept the external things and internal thoughts as moments in time that would always change. Instead, what I found to be the true foundation of my happiness was loving myself and finding that passion for life within.

At this time, I began to discover Ted Talks, the Buddhafields and Seed Festivals, and speakers like Mac Macartney, Satish Kumar, Pete and Lily from 'We The Uncivilised'. (Make your next festival a Seed or Buddhafields festival – it will blow your mind and open your heart.) All this led to a rabbit warren of research, mindfulness courses, and – dare I say it – reading. I had never been a big reader, but this was different. I was feeling inspired and curious about life. My life began to change.

This hapless carpenter got offered a gig as a part-time carpentry tutor in adult education. Stepping in front of my first class filled me with dread, but I then went on to qualify as a tutor and taught many things as well as teaching mindfulness whilst pulling from my own life experience. I was even teaching spoon-carving, a skill I picked up at Buddhafields. Who would have thought how much I would love teaching? And my career changed, to become a tutor.

After a few years, by which time I was mainly working in an office managing tutors rather than being a tutor, it was time for change again. I was beginning to relish change and the richness it would bring and I found myself in Kashmir volunteering for a few months, opening my eyes to another world ... permaculture. My return to the UK saw another change for me and I chose to spend a year living off-grid. I stayed in a shepherd's hut to experience the four seasons and nature as closely as I could.

During this time, I was picking up work back on the tools again. I found myself working with the very men I was working with years ago, an absolutely fabulous bunch of misfits. I say that from a place of love, as they really are a fine team of men. Things had changed, though. I was different.

I talked about stuff like emotions, meditations, and other shit like that. All this earned me a new nickname. There I was standing proud as 'Fat Gandalf'. A few weeks later 'Fat Gandalf' was working in a room with a decorator, a 62-year-old tattooed former heavyweight boxer – the type of chap that is good to have as a friend and not as an enemy. 'You know what Si, I am so fucking lonely, I mean I have kids and grandkids, but I go back home every night and cry. What did you do to stop this? I just want to kill myself.' So, with love, empathy and compassion I listened.

Our lunch breaks after that consisted of a few hairy-arsed blokey blokes sat round talking about emotions, feelings and neuroscience. Can you imagine the sight?

I had just met Emily, a life coach and meditation teacher, at a festival and I asked her to record a guided meditation for us about self-worth. So, there we all were, a bunch of builders meditating and their response was fabulous. One young labourer said that all the tightness and anxiety in his stomach was 'now like butterflies' and he was feeling freer than he had in years. This was the point for me that a seed was sown. It took a couple of years to germinate and grow. However, '3Monkeys Coaching' is now here, offering everyone, but particularly men, the opportunity to change internally what they see, hear, and say.

So, there we have it – my story. It feels odd sharing my vulnerability in a book. I can assure you though that for the first bit up to the mountain I am asking for no sympathy. I now love that part of my life. Let's face it, even roses need shit to grow. As for the second part where I talk about me and what I have done, I can't take the credit. We are all the same. Young, old, fat, thin, black or white, rich, poor – we are all wired the same. Never think there is a mountain you cannot climb. We all have the innate ability within us to be happy, and to grow.

Oh, and that reminds me, here's the reason why being asked to write this was inconvenient and at an extremely opportune moment: I received the email inviting me to write this as I was climbing Snowdon, this time full of life and happiness, and with my best friend, teacher, and lover, Emily. Life is about to change again; we are getting married next year. We are both passionate about coaching and believe everyone has the innate desire and will to reach their potential.

'The present moment is sometimes unacceptable, unpleasant, or awful.

It is as it is. Observe how the mind labels it and how this labelling process, this continuous sitting in judgment, creates pain and unhappiness. By watching the mechanics of the mind, you step out of its resistance patterns, and you can then allow the present moment to be. This will give you the taste of the state of inner freedom from external conditions, the state of true inner peace. Then see what happens and take action if necessary or possible.

Accept – then act. Whatever the present moment contains, make it your friend and ally, not your enemy. This will miraculously transform your whole life.'

Tolle, E. (2020) ***The Power Of Now, A Guide to Spiritual Enlightenment.*** Yellow Kite.

About Simon

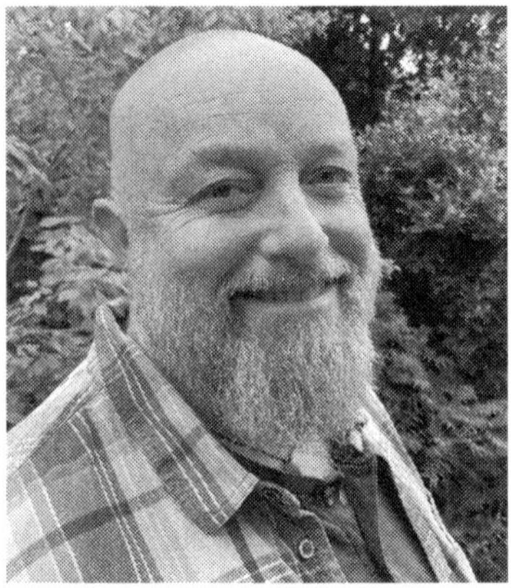

Simon Walker is a transformational life coach with a particular interest in coaching men around positive mental health and emotional resilience.

Simon has worked in the building trade as a carpenter, and owned his own company project managing the creation of exhibition stands internationally. His life's journey has taken many turns as a carpenter, project manager, and curriculum tutor developing adult education provision in the south-west of England. Simon runs spoon-carving workshops to enable a connection with nature and our human roots. He is an experienced mindfulness practitioner and teacher, and a qualified sound therapist.

Simon uses these skills and his extensive experience of the building industry, knowing how difficult it is for men to talk, to hold space for them as individuals and groups and enable them to share in a meaningful and supported way.

He lives and works with his partner, Emily, and enjoys a country walk with a pub lunch at the end of it.

You can reach Simon at:

www.3monkeyscoaching.com

Ask Better Questions

Mark Pitcher

Do you have a favourite word? I'm not sure I do. There are many words that I like but I'm not sure I have a favourite – except perhaps *mantequilla,* which means butter in Spanish. Of all the words in the world for butter, I think the Spanish say it best. I just like the sound of it. There are some words, however, that I actively dislike and top of my 'dislike list' are the words *nice*, *normal* and *fine.*

Nice because it's such a poor excuse for an adjective, when there are so many others to choose from. Maybe it's just too polite and lazy for my liking.

Normal often comes loaded with judgement and is another one that rankles. My experience is that everyone has their own version of normal and that's ok. Who are we to decide who and what is normal based on our individual perspective of the world? Certainly not me. In fact here, in 2020, aged 52, I don't believe I even know what normal means anymore.

Top of this list though has to be *fine*. Unlike words that express, tell or give us a feeling or an image, the word *fine* (in the context of feelings and emotions) tells us nothing. It is a conversation closer of a word. It is a clever disguise of a word that often hides a myriad of deeper feelings below the surface. It is a weapon, and a very effective one used by many men to deflect or shut down any attempt to get near our emotions and real feelings. It's like an old-style railway signal that flicks up to fend off any attempt to tap into our real feelings: 'Ding, ding, ding! Don't go near there!'

Intellectually many men know that there are huge benefits to making ourselves vulnerable. Men who are prepared to make themselves vulnerable often make better team members. Also, many women often cite 'vulnerability' as one of the qualities most sought after in men. However, emotionally it can be a very scary place to go. For older generations, it often goes against what we've consciously or subconsciously been brought up to believe about what it means to be a man, particularly a man in an ever increasing woman's world. So, we stick to our comfort zones instead. We talk about *what* we do and *how* we do it, but not *why* we do it or how we *feel* about it. Favourite topics are often sport, politics, work, more sport, more work – anything, as long as we don't have to talk about our feelings.

My eldest son Charlie used to say *fine* a lot. 'I'm *fine* Dad,' he would say. Sometimes I knew he wasn't but I felt powerless to break through this effective shield of protection placed before me. Without warning, Charlie took his own life in July 2016, sending a shockwave through our family. The word *fine* has since been banned in our family. One never truly gets over something like this. I am forever changed and see the world differently.

Whether I like it or not, mental health and particularly men's health (4 out of 5 suicides are still men) has been thrust front and centre into my life. I'd never considered banning anything before, especially not a word. I was pleasantly surprised therefore to read the words of Brene Brown in her fantastic book 'Daring Greatly'[1] who had done exactly that in her family by banning the words *loser* and *stupid*. Brown's work is heavily and unashamedly female-orientated and it almost pains me that such great work is lost to a male audience who need it more than ever. The world now needs, more than ever, great works such as these to be targeted at and accessible to a male audience. The world needs more real conversations, and more environments where it is normal to talk about our feelings.

So, how to penetrate and break the shield? Having re-invented myself and re-trained as a coach, I have learnt a great deal since Charlie's death. I have learnt about communication and how to engage people and 'get under the surface' more effectively. If I had to condense all of my learning into one sentence, I'd say: Ask better questions. Talking with people about their lives, their innermost thoughts, feelings and insecurities is both a privilege and a challenge.

I certainly don't pretend to have all the answers. It's one thing to do it professionally and quite another to do it effectively within your own family. However, the way a question is framed and the timing of it are important when

1. *Brown B, and White K,* Daring Greatly (Blackstone Audio 2012)

trying to open up real conversations about real feelings. Being as specific as possible, avoiding generalisations and closed questions are other tips. Making questions feel natural and well-spaced (no one likes to feel like they're being interrogated) is also good.

There's no magic formula but better questions open up better conversations. One conversation might be all it takes to save someone from themselves – to feel heard, listened to, understood. Sometimes it's the fifth time you ask a question, in a different way, that gets you to the truth, to the result. It worked for Colombo, for those of you reading this that remember him! His now classic parting question 'just one more thing…' saved up for last, and asked in a different way, would often catch his suspects off guard and achieve a breakthrough. The words you choose (we're back to words again), the order of those words and the tone of those words are all important.

Conversations though are a two-way street. So, this is where the Colombo analogy ends! Encouraging men to open up often means being brave enough to go first. Being prepared to make oneself vulnerable as one man to another man with no guarantee of it being reciprocated is scary as hell and takes courage. It's why most men don't go there. Women, it seems from experience, are much better at this than men. Why does it have to be so hard for us? This is something that needs to change and it is my hope that this book, with its wonderful stories, will go some way to changing that.

I wish I'd been braver with Charlie, been more open about my feelings, my struggles, my failures, my mental health. Maybe it would have allowed him to open up more, given him permission, moved him on from his dark place. Maybe it would have been enough to have saved him, or maybe not. Whilst I will take these thoughts and feelings to my grave, I am at the same time hopeful and positive for a brave new world in which more men can be brave enough to 'go first', where more men are prepared to push open the door and make it ok to talk about our feelings, emotions, fears and worries, without shame or fear of judgement.

It's time to lay down our proverbial shields and change this male culture and stereotype of not opening up about anything in our life because that's the point. It's not a weakness, it's actually a strength.

Here's to bringing men together in an environment that creates connection, purpose, healing and hope.

About Mark

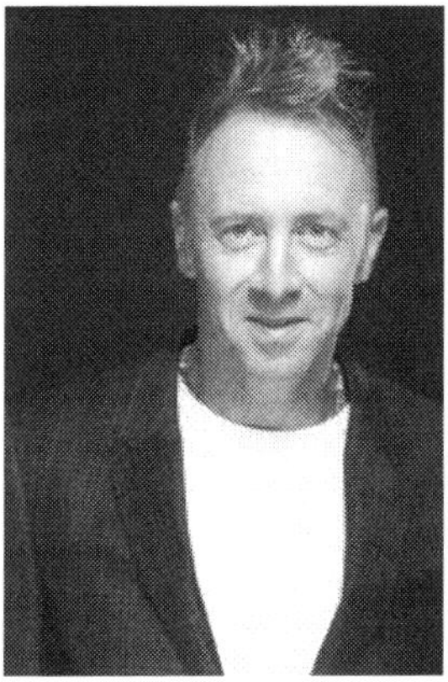

Mark Pitcher is the founder of Holistic Adventures, an offline (and sometimes online) experience that helps men and women release emotional pain and trauma. Part-holistic retreat, part-coaching workshop, part-adventure camp, the experience offers men connection, healing, purpose and escape in a safe environment. Mark is married with four children and divides his time between London, Cornwall and Barcelona.

'Dealing with emotions and trauma doesn't have to be done exclusively in a white-walled therapist's office. Getting together outdoors in nature and finding connection with other like-minded people can also help ease trauma, release stress and improve one's overall quality of life in so many areas. Allowing life to once more be an adventure rather than an endurance is possible after experiencing a trauma.'

Mark Pitcher

Connect with Mark

www.holistic-adventures.com

mark@holistic-adventures.com

www.instagram.com/markpitcher_smashthebox

www.facebook.com/SmashTheBoxMarkPitcher

Removing the Mask

Jamie Marloo Thomas

(An oral story put into writing by Sara Jones)

Preface

As an Aboriginal man, I am a storyteller with 100,000 years of an oral culture flowing through my veins. We tell stories through ceremony, singing, dancing, art and passing on knowledge from one generation to the next. We didn't and don't often write so I've asked my partner Sara to help me share my story with you by writing it down for me.

* * *

I first remember wearing a mask when I was about eight years old at school, and when the teacher asked me if everything was OK at home, I remember saying: 'Yes, everything is fine.' But it wasn't. It was anything but fine.

I grew up in a tiny country town in regional Victoria, Australia with a lot of family violence in my life. I never had my Aboriginal dad, or his family, in my life. My mum had me as a young girl – she was only 16 when I was born, but my mum wasn't ready to be an adult let alone a parent.

Mum was a teenager. She wanted to be like other teenagers, going out with friends, drinking at the pub. As a little boy, she would try to put me to bed early so she could head down to the pub. But I would know what she was up to and climb out the window to follow her, howling so much that she would finally give in and take me with her. I would fall asleep under the pool table and the publican would remind Mum to take me with her before she headed home at the end of the night.

Mum was always making jokes, stirring me up or teasing me. It was one of her coping mechanisms. She was a good teacher.

Now, as an older man, I look back and say that my mum also wore a mask. She constantly found herself in horrific family violence situations that not only impacted her body, mind and spirit but also impacted me in every possible way, and as a result I learned from an incredibly young age to hide the ugliness. Like Mum, I became the joker at school.

Whilst growing up in very small towns made it easy to hide the ugliness, there weren't enough people to care as they were either dealing with their own trauma or creating it. I was surrounded by the vastness of the bush. I would spend hours getting lost in my bush sanctuary, safe from the things and people hurting me. As an Aboriginal kid, I was connected to my birth country beyond what I could ever explain to other people.

I thought I was Mowgli out of The Jungle Book. I would literally swing out of the trees, run through the creeks and hang out with the animals who were my friends. The comfort and safety of the bush helped me to survive.

But it's not surprising that as a young boy surrounded by alcoholics, that I also found another layer to add to my mask when I started numbing my mind, body and spirit with alcohol. As a result of all the childhood abuse, I was already suffering from nightmares and chronic anxiety which later turned into full-blown depression, lasting for decades.

After running away from home at 12 to live with my beloved uncles, I was lucky enough to be involved in sport which helped me deal with the sense of worthlessness I felt as a young teenager. But when I wasn't playing sport and found myself in social settings, drinking helped me cope.

It's no wonder that my uncles encouraged me to play as much sport as possible. I would constantly be playing some sort of competitive sport, which I was a natural at, from footy to athletics to basketball. And then I found boxing.

I never knew my dad but I followed in his footsteps, and that of his dad, to become a boxer. Boxing is in the blood of my Aboriginal family – maybe because we were fighting for as much outside of the ring as in it.

When I started winning at boxing, I found that people started treating me differently. The racism eased. People wanted to hang around me. I felt accepted. I found that I was boxing more for acceptance than for me. I wanted to prove I was worthy.

I won two Australian amateur boxing titles and I was the hit of my small town. I would be given free pies and beers and my girlfriend was from one of the well-to-do families in town.

But when I decided to hang up my gloves rather than go professional, which would have meant leaving my hometown and moving to the big city of Melbourne six hours away, the racism returned and the people that I thought were friends started dropping away. I was no longer the boxing superstar. I was no longer meeting their expectations. In this despair, I learnt that if I could just keep meeting others' expectations of me, I could receive their love and approval … so I added another layer to my mask.

It was too hard to stay living in my hometown and I, ironically, made the decision to move thousands of kilometres away to the Red Centre of Australia, to the town of Alice Springs in the Northern Territory. I wanted to start the journey of finding my culture by living and working with the Arrernte people of the desert. This also began my lifelong passion for culturally mentoring boys.

All my working life, as an Aboriginal man working in community, I had jobs where people held high expectations of me and perceptions of who I was and how I should act. So when times were hard, rather than reaching out I would hide. I would tell everybody that I was okay. I would hide in my house so no one could see me drinking bottle after bottle until I re-emerged from the darkness saying I had been sick with the flu.

After three years of hiding in Alice, I decided to go home to my Aboriginal nan's traditional country in south-west

Victoria. Taking my knowledge of what I had learnt in the desert, I was thirsty to learn my own culture, seeking out elders and family to sit with to learn the 'Old Ways'. My passion grew and I started asking elders to help me revitalise these 'Old Ways', to start practising culture again, doing ceremonies, dancing and singing for country as well as learning the language. It was an amazing time of my life and it also introduced me to the concept of cultural responsibility and to pass on what I was learning to others, to keep our culture alive. Cultural responsibility added a layer to the mask that would break me.

During these years, from my early twenties, I sought help from doctors, counsellors and psychiatrists. But in doing so, I felt like a fake. I was meant to be the strong one, to be the one others turned to for support, for advice and for strength.

Working in jobs supporting Aboriginal people, I was counselling people with drug and alcohol issues, with health issues, with family violence issues, with mental health issues. Yet all along I was also suffering from these very same issues. I was suppressing my own demons, the ones I hadn't faced as a young child but which were always present.

Over the years I continued to work in these spaces, supporting and culturally mentoring people. I was really good at prioritising everyone else's needs. They found it was very easy to talk to me about such matters because I understood. I understood the feeling of worthlessness. I understood the feeling of anxiety. I understood being depressed. I understood self-medicating with alcohol.

As you grow older, you start to develop coping mechanisms – some good ones, and some not so good. The not so good ones often led me to make poor choices and bad decisions that weren't beneficial for myself or the people around me. I would then feel terrible and ashamed of myself. I would beat myself up more, only increasing my anxiety and depression.

This was a pattern that continued for decades.

But in between episodes, I was highly functioning. I did well in all my roles, helping and supporting many. I revitalised culture in my community with my elders. I culturally mentored boys and men for 26 years. I created great programmes and ran numerous camps. I even created a Cultural Foundation that gave culture and belonging to hundreds of people as well as employment. I also co-created an earth connection wellness modality based on ancient ways of knowing, doing and being.

In many ways, being highly functioning was one of my biggest problems because everyone wanted me to keep my mask on; they wanted me to keep pretending to *be fine* so that they could keep benefiting. My mask served them as much as it served me, if not more. My drinking increased trying to hide from the pressure of being me.

Then one day, my mask didn't serve anyone any more and I spiralled out of control; I couldn't have stopped it even if I had tried. Everything came crashing down around me but I didn't care anymore. I couldn't keep living with the mask – it was literally killing me.

Finally, I was able to find the courage and strength to break free from my own shame, my own fears and my own guilt. I stopped being fine and I asked for help.

It's only been 12 months since I took off the mask and showed my world who I really was.

During this time, I've really had to dig deep and explore, to re-discover who I was at the very core of my mind, body and spirit. I realised I was suffering from imposter syndrome. I was telling people how to be healthy, how to be well, how to take care of themselves and their families when in my own life I wasn't doing or being this. I wasn't practising what I was preaching. I couldn't keep prioritising other people's cultural and health needs over my own. I needed to heal me to be able to help others heal.

So the journey began to redefine and rebuild who I was as a human being of Mother Earth.

I wore the mask for so long because I was so scared people wouldn't love me if they knew all of me with all my flaws. Many of those that I gave so much to didn't stand by me so my worst fear was realised. But there were many who stayed. I'm forever grateful for the people who have stood by me, who have helped me become the person I am today.

It is truly a transformational experience hitting rock bottom. It is humbling to say to your loved ones – family and friends who time and time again have reached out to extend their hand of help in hope – that you will become a better version of yourself, that you will try to learn to love yourself.

Yes, it takes time to heal old wounds. The scars on my spirit and body will always be there but now I find myself wearing them with pride.

These scars represent my journey and the battle that I've had to go through to be a healthier, more present and connected human being. Now I find myself looking into the mirror, telling myself that I am worthy, I am lovable and that I have a purpose on this planet.

I also find myself having a little dance, smiling and celebrating this new version of myself, whom I have fallen in love with.

One thing I want to say to other men out there in a society that for centuries has told us that we need to be brave and stoic, to hide our feelings, to not cry or admit to our weaknesses ... this is so wrong for the human spirit. We need to release our fears, anxieties and emotions, to explain rather than hide them. Please reach out to family, friends and professionals before it's too late, before it eats away your very soul.

It is so important to understand as human beings that we have multiple purposes on this earth, and to find these. We must connect to each other and provide compassion, to understand where our place is in our communities and societies; finding our passion, finding our connection to that passion, and using it to better ourselves and others.

But most importantly we must connect to and become an earth steward for Mother Nature because there is no greater purpose than looking after the planet for future generations like our ancestors did before us.

I still have bad days but now I say, 'That's fine.'

About Jamie

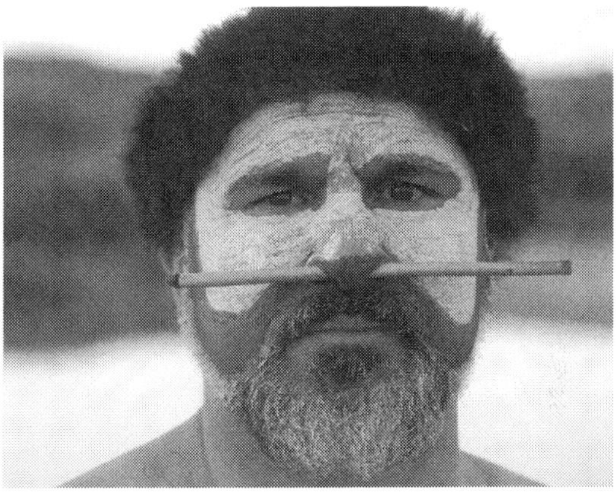

Jamie Marloo Thomas is a Senior Cultural Knowledge Holder and Storyteller for his GunaiKurnai and Maara Communities of Victoria, Australia.

Jamie is the co-founder and director of the social enterprise Wayapa Wuurrk P/L, holds a graduate certificate in Family Therapy and a diploma in Reiki. Combining over 30 years of vast professional experience in Cultural Heritage, Health and Well-being, Family Violence Prevention and Mentoring Indigenous Youth with his personal connection practice rooted in Aboriginal Dance and Ceremony, Jamie created Wayapa in consultation with Elders and Community.

Jamie is also a published author and a regular speaker at conferences and events.

In 2014, Jamie and his partner Sara Jones created Wayapa Wuurrk®, an internationally-accredited and trademarked Earth Mindfulness Connection Modality. Based on the indigenous wisdom of living in harmony with the environment, Wayapa combines ancient earth mindfulness and earth action with embodied storytelling to create Earth Mind Body Spirit Well-being.

Jamie is passionate about revitalising ancient ways of knowing, being and doing to help people to heal and create purpose, belonging and intergenerational well-being for a healthier, more connected planet.

Connect with Jamie:

www.wayapa.com

www.facebook.com/wayapawuurrk

www.instagram.com/wayapawuurrk

www.twitter.com/wayapawuurrk

www.youtube.com/channel/
UCEitY7tVyxZzbQkHK6Wis0g

www.linkedin.com/company/wayapa-wuurrk

Physician Heal Thyself

Rev. Kasey Corbin

Who knew I would become a doctor who could heal the most important person in the world, myself? Born to a single mother, in a house which my Mama still calls home to this day, into conditions of poverty in July of 1971, I made my cameo appearance on this planet. Lord knows I had no conscious clue about the energy and vibrational frequency of what I was being born into. But, as a baby, who does? I could not prepare myself for what I was about to experience, good or bad. I could only assimilate all I was to be associated with in my environment, immediate and at large.

Are you really a physician, Kasey Corbin? Well, maybe not in the traditional or academic sense of what you were taught to believe a physician is and is not. But, in the personal sense of the term, I am my own physician; no one can deny me the right to be a healer of myself, to treat myself spirit, mind and body. And, if the truth be told, you are a physician as well. Do you recall ever visiting a practising physician only to hear the classic words, '*What seems to be the problem*?' When I found the strength and courage to answer this question, it set me on the high road to self-healing later in life.

As both the physician and the patient, I posed that all-encompassing question to myself: *What seems to be the problem, Kasey*? A profound answer was revealed to me: *You are the only problem you will ever have, and you are the only solution*. Let us affirm this in the first person, present tense, to get the full impact of what you've just read. Affirmation: *I am the only problem I will ever have, and I am the only solution*. Progressively, I began to realise that I could not get better if I did not address the *It's You* issue. It is never the other person; it is you.

What? What do you mean it is never the other person? Do you know what he said? Do you know what she said? Do you know what they tried to do to me? I've heard you. And do you know that we draw or attract that which is like unto ourselves? Do you know that it is done unto you as you believe? Always. Life meets you the way you meet life. Life treats you the way you treat yourself. Someone asked me to take a dose of this elixir over two decades ago and it did not taste good. I spat it out only to have to take it again years later. It reminds me of the horrible smell and taste of that cod liver oil and castor oil my grandmothers used to give me to get better. But it worked. And this will work too.

William Shakespeare, in his play, Hamlet, Act I, Scene III, lines 78-82 wrote: '*This above all: to thine own self be true, and it must follow, as the night the day, thou canst not then be false to any man…*' To this, I would one day give heed. I now pose this question to you, the reader: *What seems to be the problem?* I would have you know that it is okay to be broken. It is okay to hurt and experience pain. It is okay not be okay. It is okay not to be fine. It is okay not to have it all together. It is okay not to have all the answers. It is okay not to be tough all the time. It is okay to fall down. It is okay to cry. It is okay to ask for help and it is okay to keep asking for help until you get it. *What seems to be the problem?*

I was stuck in the story I was born into, holding in my consciousness the self-sabotaging thoughts and feelings of hopelessness, helplessness and worthlessness. Neuro Linguistic Programming research proves that these feelings are classic signs of negative, limiting beliefs about oneself. As a self-healer, I was able to locate the information given to me surrounding my feelings of hopelessness, helplessness and worthlessness, and begin the process of restructuring the feelings by replacing the information surrounding them with empowering beliefs about myself. Let's affirm simple restructuring feelings of self-empowerment:

> **Hope** – *It's possible.* This simple affirmation gives you tons of hope.
>
> **Help** – *I can be it. I can do it. I can have it.* This is self-help, self-affirming power.
>
> **Worth** – *I deserve it.* This is self-value and self-love.

Feeling Afraid, Alone and Confused

It was a hot Friday in July of 1971 and my mother was home, pregnant and ready to give birth. She was surrounded by people who loved her and her midwife, my great aunt, my grandmother's (*father's mother*) sister called Minnie. The anticipation was great. What was she going to have? A boy or girl? I came forth out of the womb into a familial story of poverty, and poverty, like everything else, is energy and, like everything else, it has its own vibrational frequency. And, if it is ever mentally tuned in to, it can become someone's worst nightmare. And it did. Mine.

Equally, poverty can also become someone's prodding catalyst, driving force and a springboard from which to make a decision to be more, do more and have more. Sometimes I still dream about it and then I quickly change the channel. Poverty can be seen, heard, tasted, touched, smelled and felt emotionally. It has its own unique set of characteristics and qualities, the worst of which is the attitude of poverty.

As a child, when it rained outside it rained inside our house. We had a tin roof and it had holes in it. The water caused leaks all throughout our house. We used to put out buckets and pots all over to catch the water. We did not have a working bathtub or a hot water heater. We used to bathe in oversized foot tubs, and we boiled the water on the stove top in the wintertime so we could take warm baths.

There were arguments, anger and frustrations around not having enough money, wondering where the money we needed was going to come from for food and utilities. Our house was infested with roaches and mice, and it was hard to keep it cool in the summers and hot during the winters. Writing this chapter evokes so many emotions associated with the disease of poverty. Yes, it is a disease and, like all diseases, it too can be cured.

Around the age of 31, I recall holding a conversation with my Mama, a talk which brought me out of the darkness of not understanding the real motive behind why I was raised with so much pain, a dialogue which brought me into the light of an amazing '*Ah-ha*' moment – a moment I will never forget.

My Mama came to visit me one weekend while I was serving a 20-year, (actually serve 10 years), prison sentence, and I asked her, '*Why? Why Mama? I know you love me, but why did you raise me with so much anger and rage?*' With tears in her eyes she began to share with me about the emotional pain, hurt, wounds and bruises that she endured in our family lineage and from being in relationships with damaged men.

For the first time, I utterly understood that she hurt her children emotionally because of the unresolved, psychological trauma of hurt and pain (*just the pain of living*) which made its way down the line to her. Most poor black people, in the deep South where I am from, did not have any outlets of counsel, as far as I know, for mental and emotional healing. All they had in a positive light was church, and the church failed them because it did not address the psychology of the people. It acted like a psycho-tropic drug and temporarily masked the pain of life. Long story short, my Mama did the best she could with what she had been poorly and insufficiently equipped with – spiritually, mentally and economically.

Over the last 25 years of reading book after book after book, I have found that the first six years of my life were, primarily, years of mental conditioning and programming all day every day, all week every week, all month every month, and all year every year. Sadly, most of it was negative emotional treatment and negative limiting beliefs about myself. From this enlightened perception and perspective, I know now that I am not a bad person. I am powerful beyond belief. The problem came in the misinformation I was given to believe about myself.

Fixed, Pre-set Adolescent years

The formative, foundational years of my life, which I had come to accept as true, shaped my adolescent years. The validity of this set of fixed, pre-set, limiting beliefs about myself had not yet been challenged. The limiting beliefs I held as a boy to live a different story were now the controlling factors of the next phase of my experience and I had no idea. I had no idea about my place in the world. These beliefs were now the controlling factors of the next phase of my experience and I had absolutely no idea.

In short, there are simply some things in life we come to accept as true about ourselves based on the repetition of information we are exposed to … things I now separate as fact and truth.

Unbeknownst to me, my adolescent years were predetermined through a process called *mental conditioning*. You will find this kind of conditioning in the making of a slave or in the making of an inmate into a prisoner. My subconscious, automatic mind was programmed with the basis of survival to stay alive and the formation of negative habits. This would eventually pave the way for low-level living, juvenile and criminal tendencies, dishonesty, stealing, and neighbourhood or street violence. If nothing changed it would remain the formation of what was now a dismal and dark predicted future for myself.

This stage of my life is when I became a voluntary victim of the disease of drug and alcohol addiction. I had seen and heard enough to know the lifestyle of an addict. I indulged and participated in this all-too-common family and community practice. From age 12 to 15, I was introduced to everything from beer to cigarettes to marijuana to powdered cocaine to liquor to addiction. And it drove me far away from attaining any kind of academic success. By the time I was 15, I had made my first illegal drug sale in the underworld. I was weaving a cable of habit which would not be easily broken.

I am the one I have been looking for

My adolescent years shaped my early to mid-adult years with more of the same up until I was 24.5 years old. I had developed a negative consciousness and it was calcifying, becoming more and more calloused with criminal tendencies, riddled with dishonesty, lies to myself and others, and a drug and alcohol addiction which was eating away at my sanity. I was allowing it to take me down faster than a falling meteorite inside of the earth's atmosphere.

I had three children to take care of, but the addiction was not going anywhere because it was not hurting me badly enough yet. My use of drugs and alcohol were never social and it was personally shameful. I used substances to totally become another person and forget all about my responsibilities, only to get sober and have my responsibilities look me in the eye, like… *'we are not going anywhere.'*

It was a very selfish way to lead a horribly irresponsible lifestyle. I had episode after episode of not being able to remember anything about the events of getting high. I would pass out most of the time and would have to depend on other people to tell me about my God-forsaken behaviour.

It was the summer of 1995 and I had just turned 24 years old. It took for a friend to die from an overdose and for my six-month-old daughter to be brought into my addiction as an involuntary victim for me to realise I had no rhyme or reason for living. I just wanted to stay high and waste away like an atrophied bodily limb.

I had threatened to kill people, fought people, made suicidal attempts on my life, and had sexual relations with people while in an intoxicated stupor without remembering any of it. People told me about it later. I was at the end of my rope and needed healing. I somehow mustered the courage to stop, look and listen to my life's current story and own it. This and many more shameful incidents gave me the guts to seek the information I could use to heal myself.

I was not a lost cause; it was the information I was given, and the information I was *not* given about the truth of me. I am the one I have been looking for. I am the saviour I seek. *We are each responsible for all of our experiences. No one else is my rescue. I am my rescue. No one else can save me. Only I can save me.*

Personal transformation

My early to mid-adult life, aged 25–40, effectively shaped my life aged 41–49. With positive and prosperous energy vibrations I began to condition my mind to help me engage the powerful process of personal transformation. Through a series of events and experiences from 2017 to 2020, I notably attracted a spiritual family. Within this family was a support system and a life of accountability to assist me on my soul's ever-unfolding perfection of infinite potential. There is power in surrounding oneself with only quality people.

I adopted Rev. Ike as my spiritual mentor and he provided more insight about my adolescent life. My mind had been trained with thoughts and feelings of no self-confidence, no self-esteem, no self-awareness, no self-love, rejection, fear, anger, confusion, no self-identity, along with having no known purpose or sense of direction in the world. Rev. Ike and his brand of preaching introduced me to terms like self-love, positive self-awareness, self-motivation, self-identity, etc.

I have added to my physician's bag the invaluable modalities of Reiki and Energy Medicine and the Metaphysics of how to live by faith not by sight. I found a powerful affirmation which has been blessed with the insight to give my personal transformation structure: *I am a spiritual being and I live from the inside out through the power of my mind*. I have since fostered the powerful process of working with *Timeline Therapy*. Through this process, I can revisit an unpleasant area in my past and heal myself in that moment. *Life is a fight for territory. And the moment we stop fighting for what we want, what we don't want will automatically take over.* As I bring my chapter to a close, I want to answer a few questions I was asked while writing.

How did you heal from your drug and alcohol addictions?

Initially I healed from the drug and alcohol addictions out of sheer desperation and determination. Enough was enough. I was tired and I wanted to get off the merry-go-round. The pain of losing a friend to a drug overdose and the pain of making my daughter an involuntary victim of my own disease was more than enough for me to call it quits. I did not know if I could do it, but I did it. I went cold turkey. I knew nothing about detox and withdrawals. It was extremely hard and difficult ... the cold chills, the sweating, the putrid smell of the substance coming out of my pores. I have written down the process of what I did 25 years ago, and I teach it in substance abuse programmes. It is called '*Victim or Victor – the secret to overcoming addiction.*'

What role(s) do your children play in your life?

My children play the role of my 'why'. They are why I get up and do it every morning. They are the reason why I have chosen to leave a legacy and not a liability. They are the reason why I am writing this chapter. They are the reason why I will sleep in my truck if I have to. They are the reason behind my 150% philosophy.

Did you have any epiphanies while you were incarcerated?

Yes, I had a personal epiphany. Books! Reading! I found myself and I found GOD. When I found myself, I found GOD. When I found GOD, I found myself. To know myself is to know GOD; to know GOD is to know myself. I found what the systemic deception of racism tried to hide from me in books. They did not expect me to read anything about myself. What I read about myself revealed the mystery that the system had tried to keep me away from – ME. When I began to read for myself, when I began to study for myself, when I began to do research for myself, while incarcerated, the information about myself was mind-blowing. Reading saved my life and it saved me from self-destruction.

About Kasey

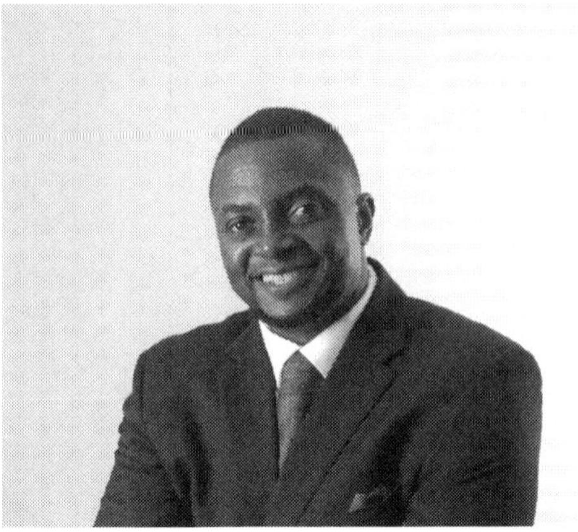

Rev. Kasey L. Corbin is a highly regarded motivational leader, thought leader, personal development coach and speaker. He is most known for his teaching ability as a seminar facilitator and for his morning spiritual broadcast called 'Wake up to the GOD in you,' a cup of morning motivation with Rev. Kasey. He has been featured on 'The Thread Wellbeing Podcast', an Australian 'Call to Rise', 'Meaningful conversations' with life coach Beata Reid, 'Let's Chai Together' with Pratibah Dey, and 'Cape to Cairo' with Peter and Anneline Coerecius' studio out of Dubai.

Rev. Kasey is known for showing the people he serves how to take possession of their minds, a quality which is required for intentional living. He has been studying the higher laws of living for the last 24 years, and for the last 13 years he has been working to help felons manage their freedom, to help inner-city residents change their self-image, to help substance abuse addicts overcome addiction, and to help young people believe in themselves.

'More gold has been mined from the mind of man than has been or ever will be extracted from the earth.'

Rev. Kasey

Connect with Kasey

www.kaseycorbin.com

www.facebook.com/pastorkaseycorbin

www.instagram.com/mountainmovingmotivation/

There's Nothing Wrong With Me

Jonnie Jensen

"There's nothing wrong with me!" I'm literally shouting in my counsellor's face. The irony of the moment painfully lost on me. "If you don't talk to your doctor about antidepressants then I will not work with you anymore," she says matter of factly. "You are unstable and you need help." I need my marriage fixing, not tablets. This is not my fault. "You can't blackmail me into taking medication."

But I can't stop seeing the counsellor. If not her then who? This is the last chance. If she can't help us then it really is over. My insides are knotted up. I'm crying. I'm angry. I'm alone. I don't want to lose my wife. "You are supposed to be helping us. Fuck you!"

It was eight weeks since I'd left. I'd hung on for way too long. I'd thought about leaving before. I could have gone quietly on my terms, done it the right way and made a positive statement, but I couldn't. I couldn't leave my two babies. I couldn't leave my wife or my marriage. My own family was all I'd ever wanted. I wasn't that guy. Yes, I was desperately unhappy, but I still loved her so much.

For years I kept telling myself it would get better. We would overcome all our troubles. It would be an inspiring story and an incredible happy ending. But who was I kidding, it wasn't and hoping it would was killing me.

It was a dark October night in 2015. Unexpectedly, after two weeks of asking, my wife agreed to talk. The conversation didn't go well. I was broken, out of control and desperate. "You don't care about me," I shouted then ran off. I head butted a wall. I ran back, shouting again, "I'm going. I'm going to kill myself. You'll never see me again." and away I stumbled into the cold, wet, evening. I didn't know where I was heading but I was certain I was going to end the heartache.

I'd thought about it enough times. It started as a random lonely thought. A possible but unlikely solution. How easy would it be? Would people miss me? What would they say? More like a conversation with myself about ways to ease the struggle. Suicide is easy. It stops the pain. It is simple.

* * *

It had been an awful 5 years. It didn't feel fair. How could one couple go through so much? We didn't deserve this. I didn't deserve this. I'd had enough to deal with when I was younger. This - my marriage, my own family - was supposed to be different.

We really couldn't have known what we were going to come home to after our honeymoon. The financial crisis had hit. It was November 2008. We arrived home to find both of us had lost our jobs.

Financial hardship puts a burden on any couple. What it also does is highlight differences between two people. We were beginning to pull in opposite directions. To me, the search for love and security was finally over. That loss felt when my mum died. When my dad had hit me. The inner turmoil and secret loneliness as a teenager. It was all over. I had my forever love. We would be fine. But we weren't.

And then came our medical challenges. Tragic experiences which put incredible strain on our marriage. I tried to look after my wife, to stay positive and keep going, but there was so little support and we drifted apart.

I kept pushing myself. Helping with the children, helping around the house, getting the shopping. I was working late into the night to make up for the days at home. I was drinking Red Bull to stay awake, watching porn to go to sleep.

All I could do was keep smiling. Keep going and hoping it would all turn out allight. But I was frantic, desperate and at times overbearing. I should have left. I know that now. I actually knew it then but I couldn't do it with two babies. They needed me and I just needed to get us through this.

By the time I was typing, "Am I burnt out?" into Google it was way too late.

The backache and headaches had become pretty persistent. They festered and niggled at my mood. I started juicing and cranked up my fitness. Always looking to fix something rather than truly resolve the big issue. And that is where the suicidal thoughts started to seep in. A fix. A solution. An exit.

I would later be told this is not normal. It is a clear sign your mental health has been seriously compromised. If you are thinking about suicide then you need help. It is that simple.

Christmas 2014 delivered the final straw. I love Christmas, all my family does. We were meeting at my brother's in Brighton to celebrate. My dad, my sister, our families and our little brother, Joe. He'd had his troubles over the last few years but they seemed to be getting better. We'd seen each other in November at a family christening. He had his own mental health struggles but thankfully he was looking well and chatting to us all. So where was he?

Come 6 o'clock it was time for us to drive home. Our babies needed their beds and so did we, but as the day rolled on Joe still had not arrived.

Shortly after returning home my brother called. "Joe is missing. His front door's open, his wallet and laptop gone. We are looking for him around Brighton."

Wow. That was tough news to take. Being an hour away there wasn't much I could do except to use my social media skills to spread the word. Between 8 pm and 2 am I sat, creating posts and images. Anything and everything in case someone had seen him. As I climbed into bed, my wife asked how it was going. "Nope. No sign." I started to pray. Calmly at first, quite traditional church-like. But then I got upset and angry.

"If you are who you say you are Jesus, then do your business now for us. Go and get my brother. It is cold, goddamn it. Do not leave him alone tonight."

Early the next morning friends, Lynne and Martin, arrived to drive me back to Brighton. I didn't register at the time but Martin lost his brother when he was younger. It was so gracious of them. As I continued my social media search, I watched out of the window as my dad taped "Missing" posters to lampposts. Surely someone knew where he was. It turned out they did. Having police in your house is a strange feeling. Time slows down. Suddenly everything echoes. I looked down the corridor at my dad. His lip quivering, "It's over", he says.

My dad and ex-step mother, certainly weren't close but for now they are hugging. I watched on as the police left. Joe took his life at a train station in East Sussex on December 29th 2014. Two weeks later I helped lower his coffin into the ground. Two weeks later I separated from my wife.

It was pretty much the hardest time of my life. I was utterly shell-shocked.

2015, as you might imagine, was not easy. That first separation was actually quite healthy. A couple of friends rallied around. I was so broken that I started talking about my upset. Lines of communication were opened and some of this upset was shared between us. Going for a walk together to talk felt like a good idea but it was actually a bad idea. Yes we needed to talk but not like that. Out of the blue on a cold, dark Sunday night. Three days earlier I made an entry in my video diary. It was the first time I had admitted to myself that the relationship was over. Not honouring my values and staying in a painful relationship was shortsighted. I was calm and measured. It made sense.

On that October night racked with blame and sorrow, my rant to my wife was anything but calm. Off I stormed. Being a Sunday there were no trains so I headed to the motorway and my way to end everything.

After twenty minutes thinking about my family, about my brother's funeral, I called my aunt. She was my mother figure. As peaceful and loving as always, she said "Stop right there. We're coming to get you". Leaning against a closed shop window, I slumped down on to the pavement. Pulling my knees in close, I cried desperately. I knew I'd lost the thing I'd spent my whole life dreaming of finding.

Breaking up from your wife was terrifying. The end of your marriage. It was not something I had a backup plan for. Where would I go? What about the kids? Money? It is a vast and empty topic. Terrifying most of all because it is the unknown. It felt like nothing would ever matter again.

By this time my depression and mental health was painfully obvious to even myself. I tried to find a counsellor. Not easy. In hindsight the obvious thing to do is ask other people if they can recommend anyone.

The first person I saw was like a stuffy school teacher. It cost me £50 for the pleasure of deciding not to work with her.

That was how I found myself back with the counsellor from the Church. It was her who insisted I needed antidepressants and she wasn't going to work with me if I didn't take them. Which was how I finally ended up at the doctors. A meeting that I should have had about four years earlier.

"You know you have every right to be depressed. It is a medical condition," explains the locum doctor I'd never seen before. "You have been through an incredible series of emotionally stressful situations. You are depressed. Your answers and tears show me that. There is no shame. It is just time to get you better."

The doctor went on to explain what antidepressants do and how they could help me. I had nothing to lose. I certainly couldn't feel any worse.

Dealing with depression alongside a divorce was unbelievably difficult.

The path I took to get better has become the foundation for my Team Super Dad community and Hero Academy programme. At least this experience has blessed me with the knowledge to help other dads live the life they desire, not the life they feel stuck in.

I got wise about taking the citalopram tablets. From five milligrammes I went up to ten, then twenty, then forty. I read about other people's experiences, good and bad. Along with taking the highest amount prescribed I became a regular at the gym and swimming pool. Because my wife had the car, I was also cycling about eight miles a day. I was literally sweating out the sadness.

I chose to not watch any news or negative TV, which meant that I was replacing the sadness with laughter, knowledge and encouragement. YouTube, Netflix and Audible are full of it. I was literally reprogramming my mind.

A mum of an old friend recommended a counselling service, connected to a charity. They were wonderful, warm, supportive and generous. I'll never forget Julie. For eighteen months she listened and steered me to unexplored corners of my heart. Places that were still hurting from loss and loneliness in my youth. It was no wonder I hung on so tightly to relationships that didn't really work. Why I overcompensated for others and loved so unconditionally. Finding the right counsellor is a game changer.

I also joined a community singing group, where I not only found I could sing, but I also made new friends.

I took antidepressants for just under a year. I made the decision that I would not need them after that. At least that was the hope. About eight months in, I was sitting in my new home, watching TV. I became aware of how calm I was but also how detached my thoughts were from the programme I was watching. I knew, at that moment, it was time to start coming off them.

It was September 2016 and I still had a long way to go but I was back in control of my mind. I was slowly beginning to find reasons to be hopeful and look forward to a happy future, with my children, and one day a beautiful wife.

* * *

My advice to you is to be good to yourself. Be honest with the man in the mirror and don't be afraid to ask others "do you think I'm ok?".

It is not selfish to look after yourself if it means you are better able to look after the people you love most.

About Jonnie

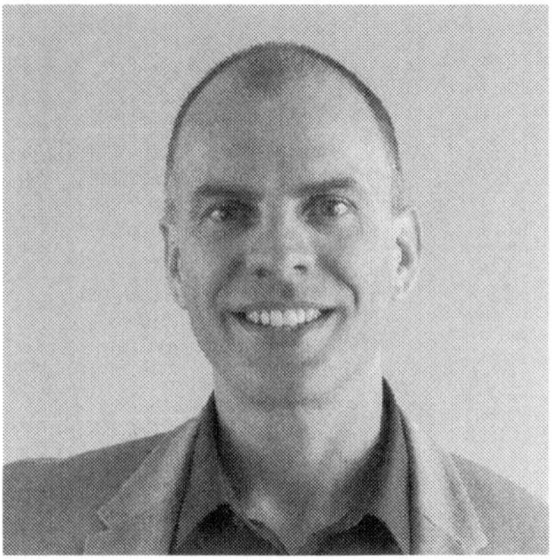

Jonnie Jensen is the founder of TeamSuperDad.com, a community and success system for dads who want to be fit, focused and successfully leading their family. Having previously worked in digital marketing for 20 years, Jonnie was inspired to create Team Super Dad after his marriage breakdown and the challenges he experienced rebuilding his life.

Jonnie lives in Maidstone, Kent, England but also considers Chicago his home after spending many happy months visiting family there. He is a father and brother with two children. As well as a passion for fitness and well-being, Jonnie is a certified fire-walking instructor. His ambition for Team Super Dad is to see dads confidently fulfilling their potential and living the life they desire, not the life they feel stuck with. He loves hosting the Team Super Dad podcast and is always on the lookout for great guests with an adventure to share.

Connect with Jonnie

www.linkedin.com/in/jonniejensen

www.facebook.com/JonnieJensen

www.teamsuperdad.com

www.facebook.com/teamsuperdad

Team Super Dad Podcast:

www.podfollow.com/teamsuperdad

From Suicide to Success

Rob Goddard

In 2010, I was on the 125th floor of the world's tallest building, the Burj Khalifa tower in Dubai, preparing for my death. For months I had searched the internet looking for painless ways to kill myself. I decided on jumping from a great height. I calculated that it would only take me 13 seconds to fall nearly 3,000 feet. Then it would all be over. It could be even sooner than that as I had read that I was likely to have a heart attack on the way down. No more pain, nor struggling, just nothing.

Just two years earlier, I was in the top 1% of earners in the UK. I was 45 years old and in the prime of my life. I had a lovely home, wife and twin boys, and I was highly successful in business. I felt invincible in life, like I was made of granite rock.

However, in a three-month period during the summer of 2008, my life crumbled. I lost my marriage, my children and my job. I went into an emotional tailspin. I fell out of the sky like an eagle that had been shot by an unknown sniper from the ground. I had never been out of work in my life and as a result I felt like a complete failure in life because I couldn't provide for my family. The centre of my world had been my career and the materialism that surrounded it. I was in a complete state of shock and bewilderment.

Extreme anxiety set in which led me to stop sleeping or eating at all for days. My mind was in perpetual turmoil trying to process what had happened and how I could sort the whole mess out. I would stare at the TV screen for long periods and not remember what I had just watched. The only thing that filled my waking and non-waking hours was the constant, torturous churn of my disastrous situation.

The day I lost my job I went to see my doctor to get some medication to help me get through this shock. In her office, I broke down. In floods of tears and broken sentences I managed to get out that I had come to the end of my life and didn't know where to turn. She was empathetic and promised that a counselling service would contact me. Then she handed me a bewildering and colourful array of pills. I thought to myself, 'Once the drugs take effect, I'll be back to my normal self within a couple of weeks and then I can start to rebuild my life again.'

I didn't know that what lay ahead of me was a five-year battle with depression and me repeatedly feeling that suicide was the only way out. Fortunately, I did meet an 'angel' and I'd like to introduce you to him later.

My situational depression was like a black menacing cloud. It came and went as it wanted for many years, affecting my emotions and my mind. I didn't talk to anyone about it; I was too ashamed of feeling the way I did. So, I just put on a brave face, a mask, to the outside world. Contrary to what you may think, it's not suicide that kills, it's the loneliness and isolation. Here's the dichotomy: in a highly connected modern world, we can isolate ourselves so easily. Most depressed people don't want to be a burden on others. Instead, they just suffer in silence, and some, in desperation, sadly take their own life.

Did you know that 2,200 people commit suicide on this planet every day? That's up 40% over the past two decades! Of those, 75% are men. Many men are far worse at expressing their feelings than women. We often lock things away, don't speak up and sometimes the dam breaks. We have a global crisis on our hands. Suicide is the biggest killer of people aged under 45 in the UK. I would have been one of those statistics had events not gone a different route.

By 2010 my life hadn't bounced back; I was still being prescribed drugs by the doctor, but by then I had started to self-medicate with alcohol. Vodka was a quick way of making my mind go fuzzy for a few hours so that I could forget my depression, albeit temporarily. Eventually I stopped taking the prescribed drugs and started stockpiling them instead. In the end I had over 700 pills tucked away in my wardrobe – a secret stash. I thought that if I couldn't control what happened in my life anymore, at least I could determine when and how my life ended. At least I had that control remaining in my life.

Because of regular anxiety attacks, I had numerous restless nights, tossing and turning like a ship caught at sea in an unforgiving storm. I started waking up later. I would keep my dressing gown on throughout the day. I didn't eat properly, didn't shave and rarely washed. I must have stunk! I had become a functioning alcoholic.

Self-employment was forced upon me – I had no choice. I did manage to slowly build a small business, but it was very tough. I remember travelling to sales pitch meetings with music blaring out of the car's speakers, crying my eyes out en route, only to discreetly park around the corner from the offices, wipe my eyes and my nose, then put on my mask. I also had a stash of mints in the car to mask the smell of vodka, which I popped before entering the building. I became an 'actor' for a couple of hours.

But life just bumped along the bottom. I was just surviving and definitely not thriving. Then, out of the blue, my main client terminated our contract and my life again spun immediately out of control. Once again I looked at the dark abyss opening up in front of me.

A Fresh Start

So, in March 2010, I decided to run away to the bright and alluring lights of Dubai to become a financial adviser, with an invitation to a job that would provide untold riches for me, or so they promised. In reality, it was a commission-only job, working in a part of the world I have never been to and in a culture which I had never encountered previously. It was an opportunity to prove to myself once again that I could bounce back. I had worked in financial services for three decades; I believed I could really do it, again.

Initially, I was so full of energy, enthusiasm and renewed hope when I went to see my new regional director at the glitzy Dubai Marina. He was half my age but had been in the country for four years and was the top salesman in the company. He had a boat in the Marina and a Porsche 911. At last, a blank canvas, a fresh start where nobody knew me. It may have been commission-only and living in one of the most expensive cities in the world, but I was up for the challenge.

I started my new job with no data, no client base, no website, no marketing budget; it was just me and a bunch of business cards and a winning smile! I figured that my target market included expatriates, high-net-worth individuals who paid no tax and were dripping with surplus cash. So, I decided to go where they tended to hang out, to meet them, chat and make myself visible. Places like the Yacht Marina, the Irish pub Fibber's McGee, The Polo Club and the prestigious car dealerships like Ferrari, Lamborghini, Porsche, and even the Harley Davidson dealership. I also used LinkedIn, creating a stream of articles on hot topics of interest to some of the world's richest people, positioning myself as a 'thought leader' in all matters financial. Leads started to flood in, new clients were signing up and at last I was making some serious money again.

However, I had completely underestimated trying to fit in with an immensely fast-moving society and what seemed, to me at least, a superficial and uncaring environment – a microclimate where people rarely had the time or inclination to build real friendships. At the same time, I had also cut myself off from my family and my close friends, working in a country 3,500 miles away.

The blazing summer sun was like an inferno and, coupled with the stifling humidity of Dubai, it was like working in my own hell. I felt like a prisoner condemned to a life of hard labour, paying for my heinous crimes. The money wasn't bringing happiness at all, and I was gradually feeling alone in the metropolis, isolated from family and close friends. It was a prison of my own making, albeit a golden one.

I gradually sunk into what felt like quicksand. The more I struggled against it, the more I got sucked into it. So, I kept what I called a 'death diary', which was me journaling about my innermost thoughts, fears and anxieties. It helped to write things down, but the main aim was to leave something behind for my children, so they would know why their dad had killed himself. I didn't want them to blame themselves or think they could have done something to change the situation.

After months of battling on my own, I eventually gave up the fight. I was emotionally exhausted and battle-weary, so I decided to go to the daunting and imposing tower of the Burj Khalifa, to find my way outside to jump. I was 13 seconds away from ending the pain and private hell that had become my life.

I woke up one morning and decided that today would be the day this torment would end. I showered and shaved like any normal day. I then phoned a work colleague and said that I wanted to visit the Burj Khalifa and take some pictures from the top of the tower because, despite working in Dubai, I never had time to do the tourist thing. I never disclosed to him my plan because I didn't want him to talk me out of it.

I met him at the front entrance, bought the tickets and joined the snaking queue of sightseers making their way to the lifts. As we travelled the 90 seconds to the top I recall having this macabre thought that it would only take me 13 seconds to come back down. I was calm, not stressing about what I was about to do. It was a surreal frame of mind to be in, having made the decision to end my pain. I felt empowered somehow to be taking control of my life.

We got to the 125th floor and wandered around the viewing platform with a multitude of tourists. I asked my friend to take some pictures of me looking out at the Dubai scenery and then excused myself to go to the bathroom. I told him I wouldn't be long. Instead, I went around the tower looking for a way to the outside of the building. The viewing platforms had thick, floor-to-ceiling, glass so I had to find an exit that workers would have used to gain access to the outside of the tower.

I quickly found a fire exit and tentatively tried the handle. It was locked! Who on earth locks a fire exit door? Someone had locked this one and so my attempt at suicide that day had been thwarted. I went back to my apartment, dejected, miserable and angry with myself. The stockpile of more than 700 tablets looked more appealing.

A Call for Help

I'm not sure why, but I decided to call a friend of mine back in the UK. Alex and I had met at a business networking event just at the time I had first gone self-employed. There was an immediate connection between us and over a couple of years we had become good friends. He was and still is a business coach and, crucially, was the only person who kept in regular contact with me after I left for Dubai. He contacted me on a regular basis to see how things were going. I looked forward to our chats, although I didn't really share the full picture. I just tried to be upbeat.

But, following my thwarted suicide attempt earlier that day, I offered to fly him out to Dubai for a few days, so that we could speak in person and at length. To my surprise he jumped on a plane and we sat poolside at my apartment for hours on end. We also laughed incessantly. It was fun sharing time together. He also told me off when he peered in my fridge and challenged me with *'I can't see anything green, only meat and alcohol!'*

Alex asked me one question that changed the direction of my life. He asked, *'What do you **really** want to do with your life Rob?'* Immediately, I said that I didn't know. But not put off by that, he persisted with, *'but if you did know, what would it look like?'*

What a great question. I then began to describe what I saw and said that I wanted to go back to my first love of mergers and acquisitions. With more prodding, visualising and planning a potentially happy future, I subsequently made the decision to return to the UK to start again.

I went on to envisage that by 2020 I would create a business worth more than £5 million, move somewhere in the Southern Mediterranean and teach English to children from a double-decker bus, and with the woman of my dreams.

With renewed hope and a clearer vision, I managed to pitch and secure 14 investors for my new business venture.

I was then able to afford to pay myself a salary for the first time in three years. It's not been easy building a business from nothing, but with unwavering determination, that fledgling business has now grown into a multi-million-pound company across two continents, employing 25 people.

Nevertheless, I still had to kill a few ghosts from the past, so three years ago I set up a sister company in Dubai. The first time round in Dubai I was a beaten man, but now when I come out of the airport terminal I have a smile back on my face in a country that so nearly became my last resting place. Initially, I was apprehensive and unsure if I could make a business work out there, having previously failed. However, I felt much stronger than before. Because the UK business had some success, I used that as my confidence platform for the new Dubai business.

Over the years I have learnt from my mistakes of the past and have surrounded myself with trusted people that I can share myself with, people who act as a sounding board, both in business and on a personal level. I've also set out to employ people who are better than me at things. There is a freedom in having others run the business day to day. That is what enabled me to get precious time back. I now own four businesses and don't work full-time in any of them!

Retirement has allowed me to do the things I want with the people I want to work with. I've broken the walls of that golden prison and have been teaching clients to do the same for the past ten years. I now help business owners find an exit strategy – closing one chapter in their lives and starting a new one. That's been my journey and I want to share with others how liberating that is. I also invest in other people's businesses and take on a few private clients for mentoring assignments. I have the privilege of being asked to speak at a wide range of other people's events, both in the UK and in the Gulf.

The Road Forward

Looking back, my resilience – the strength I found to fight back and triumph over adversity – came from speaking and sharing with others. Today I know there's no point in running away. Even in the darkest hour, it's healthier to just face up and reach out in dark times.

My relationship with money has changed too. In fact, I'm in the process of setting up a charity in order to embark on a ten-year plan to create a 'living legacy', an altruistic journey to make a difference to other people's lives through a multitude of charitable causes for those in need.

My family has expanded: I now have six children ranging from the age of 25 down to 6, with two sets of twins in that beautiful tribe! Had I been successful in my suicide attempt, I would have robbed all of them of a future with their father.

I would also never have gotten together with Kristina, the woman of my dreams, either. She is originally from Albania and we have a second home there on the beach overlooking the Mediterranean Sea. We've bought a boat too and still plan to buy that double-decker bus soon.

Retirement to me is being able to do the things I choose to do, with the people that I want to be with. I can't wait for this ten-year vision to unfold: building a charitable foundation with the woman of my dreams, and experiencing the joy of making a difference in life.

One final thought. If you are struggling right now and if you are in a dark, cold place, I urge you to find an 'Alex'.

Specifically:

Speak up and ask for help. You will **not** be a burden on anyone. Don't let isolation win. Make that call now to a trusted person. They will be honoured that you have shared something so personal with them and that you trust them.

Don't believe the lie in your head that the world would be a better place without you in it. Dozens of people will be devastated by you taking your own life and that will affect them for the rest of their lives. Suicide is a long-term solution to a short-term problem.

Alternatively, if life is ok for you, consider becoming an 'Alex' to someone that you suspect is going through a hard time. Go for a coffee or lunch and give them time and space to open up. Let them know you are there for them, any time, any place. Give them your listening ear, not instant fixes. You could be that one person they need to help turn things around. There is no better feeling to know that you have been instrumental in saving someone's life; just ask my friend, Alex.

About Rob

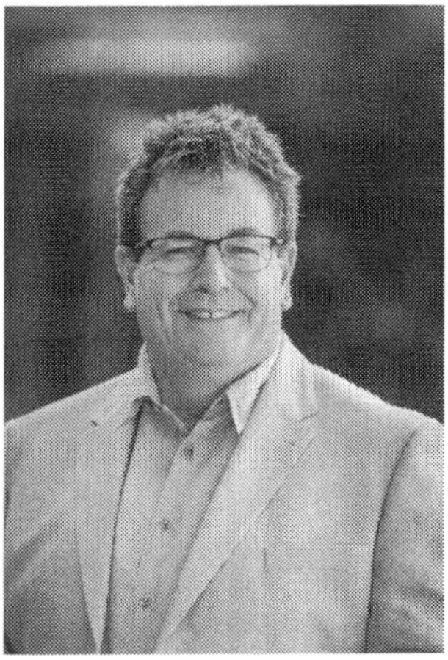

Rob now owns four businesses and has transitioned from an operator to investor, a journey many entrepreneurs struggle to make. He has trained over 6,000 business leaders and brings over 35 years of experience helping business owners finish one chapter in their lives and start a new one.

His original and largest business, EvolutionCBS Ltd, is a highly successful multi-million pound advisory firm in the UK and UAE, and since 2002 Rob has been responsible for the sale of nearly 400 privately-owned UK businesses, totalling over £2 billion in transaction values.

Rob also works on more philanthropic and altruistic projects and causes, especially in the area of depression and suicide. His signature talk, 'Suicide to Success', is a very personal story of his own battle with depression, leading to a suicide attempt, then fighting back to win and triumph over adversity, to lead a fulfilling life, filled with fun.

Connect with Rob

www.robgoddard.co.uk

rob.goddard@robgoddard.co.uk

www.linkedin.com/in/robgoddard

Buy Rob's book

www.amazon.co.uk/dp/1916220401/ref=rdr_ext_tmb

Denial to Divinity

Maria Adriana Contreras

And the mist of BEING FINE was sprayed across the land

And everybody hurt

And everybody cried

And everybody fell into a deep slumber of forgetting

And everybody carried on BEING FINE.

I have been interested in how to reduce or end human suffering all of my life. As an energy-sensitive person who empaths others' emotions like a sponge, I have been on the receiving end of much abuse on all levels. This has often left me asking the question, 'How can the rage from a person be transformed such that they stop attacking me?'

I was born into a genocide war in my native Chile. My father was tortured and killed. At the age of six my mother, my brother and I came to England as refugees. Not having the faculty of language to express my repressed feelings, things got buried so deeply that I have only truly met them and myself in recent years.

Six years ago I totally loathed myself despite being a loving kindness coach at the time. Funny, I know, and I do appreciate the adage, 'we teach what we need to learn'. Such was my intent on learning the holy grail of totally loving myself no matter what happened that the right teacher came into my path. I discovered self-love spiritual teacher Matt Kahn and learnt from his YouTube videos on a daily basis. I can now say that I love and respect myself completely no matter what life throws at me.

The greatest learning I had was that we experience the most uncomfortable, painful and destructive feelings because of denial. This is a term that is kicked about a lot in psychology, psychoanalysis and all manner of therapy. I was aware of it, however...what does denial really mean?

In Tarot, which I love as a form of storytelling and the human condition, the Death card also means denial. When there is denial there is spiritual death because no oxygen, light or goodness can pass. They are blocked, locked up and buried to good riddance.

Denial causes the greatest emotional pain. The word emotion comes from the Latin word 'emotus' which means energy in motion. Energy that is blocked due to denial therefore cannot circulate. The flow state of energy becomes trapped – a bit like having a huge amount of wind and not being able to fart. Imagine that for a lifetime. Yes, it's emotional constipation which made my guts hurt just writing it.

It made sense for me to release this energy blockage, which was both physically and emotionally painful, but how?

The spiritual or wellness coach or mentor would advise to 'just let it go' or 'forgive' which I find challenging. Trying to 'let things go' ironically made me feel worse not better and doubly worse because I'd forked out money and time to be told that I was not doing it right and needed to 'let go'.

The thing is, to get out of denial what is truly needed is something more akin to an ego death. This looks like surrendering what I perceive and dropping into 'what is'.

This sounds amazing but in practice it is a very big stretch.

What it takes is not having much of an attachment to my sense of who I think I am. So unless you've been on a solid and honest journey of self-actualisation it's a high mountain to climb. In fact it would be easier to climb a big fat physical mountain because an ego death is extremely emotionally painful. I refer to it as a 'death' because it means laying aside who I think I am. And this is a construct that is very deeply ingrained – like a massive grass stain on your trouser knee on a pair of white trousers, or worse. I know that to try to 'let something go' is a spiritually violent act and disrespectful to my soul.

I have tried for decades to let things go and relax into this surrender process. However, when I do my inner child does not like me and I come into an inner conflict. She says things like, 'You have no idea how much pain I am in, and now you are asking me to drop it?' Then she'll retreat and bury herself even deeper into denial.

The real reason that I believe challenges happen is in order to evolve and learn from them. This requires the deepest respect and dignity in my relationship with myself.

So, instead of asking for the impossible, 'just let go', I offer the opposite strategy which for me works 100% of the time. Tell us: what is the holy grail of this getting out of 'denial' jail free card?

It is not to try to get out of it, but rather to rest in it, sit with it, afford it the dignity and respect it's been asking for. 'It' being the denial has only ever been waiting to be respected and acknowledged as it is, not how I would have it be. 'It' being the denial wants to be seen as it truly is, in all its ugliness and viciousness – in its raw, unapologetic expression of un-love.

This is the point at which most soul adventurers will be too afraid to proceed because the ill feeling has been denied for a lifetime or perhaps more because is absolutely unbearable. I make no bones about it; it's horrific and any way out of it seems like a better option than to face it eye to eye.

What makes it a billion times tougher is the social, spiritual, religious, cultural, generational and gender conditioning of 'put up with a situation that is unacceptable, get over yourself, be tolerant, forgiving and say that you're fine' instead of admitting that you don't like it and do not choose it.

It is this programming of how we 'should' be that is the biggest problem. Without all of the rules, programmes, conditions, contracts and compliance training we could all be more free or – I would suggest – totally free.

I know that awakening to your true real self is simply a case of being released of all of these societal constraints.

Alright, so now to the actual solution that I have test driven and that works for me because if it didn't then I wouldn't have survived my hideous life which I can now afford to laugh about.

The problem: all types of social conditioning that have everyone locked up in the denial prison called 'being fine'.

The solution: awaken from the aforementioned dark programmes and meet your true real self that was always free.

But how?!

Three weeks ago I had the mother of all awakenings. Something happened to me that I've been trying to achieve for decades, but I do believe in natural timing. When things are ready, they happen. Such is nature's way. What happened is that in the most natural and gentle way I became open and aware of an extreme amount of unconditional love which feels like support, comfort and guardianship.

'What the bleep caused that to happen?', asked a close friend. I explained that I had been smashed so hard and into so many tiny pieces that it felt like the old Maria was truly laid to one side. And what arose from the painful and smouldering rubble was the phoenix rising from the ashes. My true light was made visible to ME.

And from this place of oh-my-god-what-the-f-just-happened was this constant connection to unconditional love. I know, right?! I'm still awed by it and don't know what to do with myself but the creativity, love, compassion and energy is off the chart and I feel like I'm vibrating off the surface of the earth.

Amazing what lockdown challenges create...

So from this place of having this 'Goddess Hotline' connection to answers that are definitely not from 'me' I am able to access a far higher intelligence. And I know that everyone has this access.

And then, just this morning as I was writing this chapter I was helping a friend with the age-old challenge of humanity, how to stop feeling really so shit, and this is what came through. It's nothing I don't already know but the way it is dreamily woven is nothing short of divine.

To move from denial to divinity follow these simple steps:

When you know something, you know it. Nobody can convince you otherwise because this is your own lived experience.

When something is hurting from what is possibly the denial of its existence, this is probably due to trying for so long to be fine and not to be affected by it.

Do the opposite.

And allow yourself to fully sense and know its presence.

Do the opposite.

And connect with it fully, as though you were looking it in the eye – being to being. But it feels horrible, horrific and hellish and you want to run, escape or say that you're fine!

Do the opposite to deny its existence.

Allow yourself to feel really horrible and fully allow the feelings to be known.

Here's the biggest key to the kingdom:

You are allowed to not enjoy every single minute of it. You're allowed to fully express whatever that thing makes you feel. This is to embrace and get out of denial.

It's the hero's journey because the faint-hearted won't be able to power through it. The intensity of the negative emotion is almost too much to bear. But therein lies the answer, because just underneath this is the light – your light. It was there all along, but who knew?

All that life of being fine and nobody was ever the wiser. So we use addictions, avoidance, denial and over-working, over-achieving and over-eating.

This is the radical path of radical honesty. Acknowledge whatever is there with dignity and respect. Look, look, look and don't look away. When 'it' is fully seen it will feel seen and take its leave. That's when 'it' lets go of you, not the other way around.

Because its job is done. Its voice has been heard. Its pain has been felt. Its ugliness has been seen.

But this is not a process that can be thought through. The mind, due to so much conditioning and mind control, does not have the full faculty of discernment which is why it is referred to as the 'monkey mind'.

Please know that it's not that we are all stupid monkeys with no control over our minds. What if we have all been coaxed into believing what is not ours?

This adventure has nothing to do with your mind, logic or thinking processes. This is about your 'knowing'. There is a part of you that knows. Your knowing comes from your journeying and adventuring and nobody can take this away from you.

Beliefs are like swords; they cause so much damage because they sway the tree from here to there in the gale-force wind. But knowing is like the tree trunk rooted firmly into the earth, like an ancient oak.

Get out of denial by knowing what you know. Put aside everything that you have been told, taught, trained in and made to believe. Hear what you know. Know what you know. It's yours and it's your wisdom.

When you know something, nobody can deny it or take that knowing away from you. This is how to undo conditioning. Your knowing is yours and you know. This is restoring your dignity back to you. This is you hearing your own truth. Your own knowing is your truth. What you know is what is true for you. Your knowing is your superpower. So sit with this knowing.

Your knowing is your access to divinity.

You are sovereign.

You are the light of awareness.

I bow to your greatness.

I honour your light.

Thank you for being here.

About Maria

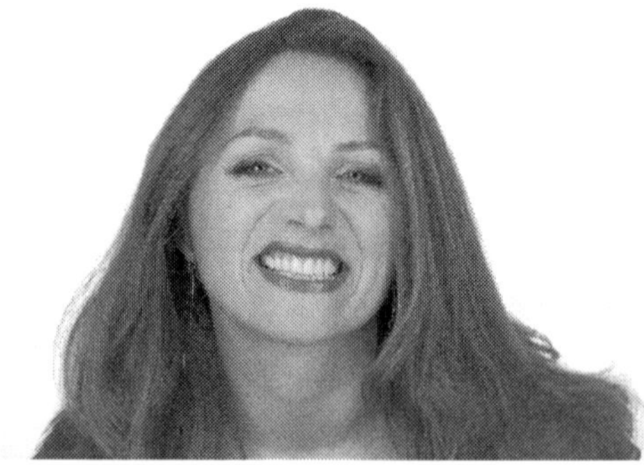

Maria Adriana Contreras is from Chile. Following the loss of her father to the dictatorship regime she was exiled with her family to England.

She is a conflict resolution specialist and leadership trainer and creator of **Body Intelligence** – somatic leadership training system.

Her powerful presence enables people to relax into their real selves and share what they are truly here to do.

Her mission is to be in true service to humanity.

Connect with Maria

www.mariaadriana.co.uk

www.bodyi.co.uk

www.linkedin.com/in/soulleadershipmentor

Through Adversity Comes Strength

John Watson Allison

It was 1991. I'd been on an arduous expedition on the island of South Georgia in the Antarctic, living on the glacier for several weeks and enduring some of the worst weather I'd ever experienced. Despite the conditions and nearly being buried alive it was an incredible adventure and one that I wouldn't have missed for the world. Of course, we're waking up now to the fact that moving beyond our comfort zone is where the magic happens. As humans we need to be challenged in order to grow.

We had a four-day boat journey on board Royal Fleet Auxiliary (RFA) Diligence, travelling from South Georgia to the Falkland Islands where I was based on a four-month deployment with the Royal Engineers. As she slipped away from the Antarctic I was able to lie back in my bunk and reflect on the many incredible lessons I'd learnt during the expedition. The four-day journey proved to be uneventful; even the seas were relatively calm and we were soon docking in the Falklands at Mare Harbour.

As the stevedores were securing the vessel, there was suddenly an announcement over the ship's tannoy: 'Could Sapper Allison report to the Captain'. It's not often that a young sapper (a private soldier in the Royal Engineers) is summoned to see the highest ranking officer onboard ship so it was with some trepidation and excitement that I approached the door of the bridge. As soon as I walked in I could see that the Captain looked a little uneasy. He handed me a piece of paper and said, 'I'm very sorry'. I unfolded the telex sheet and struggled to comprehend what I was reading. Marked 'STAFF IN CONFIDENCE, COMPASSIONATE', I was informed that my brother had passed away on 6 November 1991 and that I was to contact my father ASAP. I was in shock and it didn't seem real.

I later found out that the South Georgia expedition leader had been made aware of my brother's death before we departed the Antarctic island and had decided that it would be prudent to inform me of his passing when we docked in the Falkland Islands and not during the voyage. It was the right thing to do as there was little that could have been done while in transit in any event.

The Captain allowed me to call home on the satellite phone from the bridge of the ship. It was heartbreaking to hear the emotion in my mother and father's voices and at that moment it hit me hard. Although Clive had been my half-brother and much older than me, I'd looked up to him and considered him my brother. After I'd come home from my first experience of war, the Gulf War, Clive had come to visit me and I remembered showing him my videos of the experience. I felt we'd really been able to bond. Sadly that was the last time I saw him.

Having arrived back in the Falkland Islands and having completed the expedition on South Georgia, a few of us were heading to the bar in the Mount Pleasant military complex that night. As we downed a few pints I remember thinking that it was strange as I didn't feel anything. I had decided not to mention my brother to other Royal Engineer mates who were unaware of his passing. I felt emotionless and two days later the military flew me home. I have to say that the Ministry of Defence were amazing in dealing with compassionate cases and I couldn't fault their approach.

When I arrived home is when it really hit me again. There were reminders of Clive in the house and when I saw those I burst into tears and all the emotion came flooding out. A week later I was re-joining my unit and flying back to the Falklands. When I was back with the lads and cracking on with our tasks, it was almost like nothing had happened. In effect I was becoming adept at putting things in boxes and burying them.

Fast forward several years to 2002. My mother had been feeling unwell for a period and the GP went on to prescribe half an aspirin daily. Her health didn't improve and ultimately she was told that it was cancer of the liver. We were all stunned; my mother never smoked, barely drank, exercised regularly and was an ambassador for healthy and modest living. In an attempt to tackle the cancer head-on, my mother's surgeon attempted to operate and remove it. While she was in theatre my father and I faced an anxious wait at home, waiting for a call from the hospital.

The phone rang and my father was speaking to the surgeon. Evidently the tumour was too big to remove safely so the only option was chemotherapy. It was a huge blow but we all tried to remain positive and do the best we could to support her and help her pull through. The chemotherapy turned out to be incredibly aggressive; it was heartbreaking to see such a destructive effect on someone you love.

At the time I was serving in Northern Ireland with the Army and would fly back regularly to support her and my father. When I was back in Northern Ireland I felt like I was far removed from the situation. On reflection, it also felt like I was putting things in boxes and burying them again. Surrounded by military and police friends and doing a job I loved, I felt emotionless.

One day I flew back into Leeds Bradford Airport, picked up a hire car and drove off to Sheffield Hospital where my mother was being treated. As I headed down the motorway and got closer to Sheffield I was suddenly aware of this incredibly powerful wave of emotion sweeping over me. It was so powerful that I had to pull over into a lay-by. Suddenly all the emotion and sadness that I had been suppressing and burying exploded in floods of tears. I wanted to pull myself together and be strong for my mother and father so as soon as I had regained my composure I headed on down the motorway.

My mother was eventually moved to the Retford Hospice. I'd never really told her that I loved her so I made a point of telling her. She said, 'Of course, I know that.' As I held her hand with my father and I by her bedside, I could feel her life switch off. Judith Althea Allison passed away in March 2002.

Again, the military were amazing and my bosses Steve and Jim were incredibly supportive too. I was given compassionate leave and then eventually returned to Northern Ireland. It was easy for me; I could go back to my work in Northern Ireland. My father had to deal with an empty house and the ever-present reminders of my mother, his wife.

Having served for 24 years in the British Army and having joined at 16, straight from school, I decided that it was time to try something new. I officially left the Regular Army on 16 January 2012. What followed was a mix of adventure, academic study and holiday. I ended up living on the tiny Mediterranean island of Gozo for five months before returning to the UK in December 2012.

In 2013 I was trying to find my way in civilian life proper. Prior to that I'd completed my MA at City University, London, and then had a long sojourn in the sun. In 2013 it was time to get serious and work out what I wanted to do with my new life. On reflection, what followed have been some of the hardest years of my life. I am blessed to have had an amazing mother and father. My father is an inspiration, still walking six to eight miles a day at the age of 89, and has mastered IT like he was a teenager.

Thanks to him, we had remarkable family holidays and a very comfortable home. Army life wasn't always easy but generally I was in my element and would do it all again in a heartbeat. I'd also encourage others to do the same. I had some life-changing experiences and met some incredible people too. I always knew from a very early age that I'd join the Army. My grandfather owned a house called Brook Manor (believed to be the basis for Baskerville Hall in Sherlock Holmes, Hound of the Baskervilles) on Dartmoor, with 150 acres of woodland. I was always exploring the old copper mine tunnels in the grounds, swimming in the river, building dens and shooting my air rifle. Army life felt like my destiny. I'd gone from making homemade fireworks as a kid, to bomb disposal and latterly weapons intelligence with the Army. The pinnacle of my career was the moment when I debriefed a former Iraqi Intelligence Service bomb-maker in Baghdad and he was drawing circuit diagrams of the devices he'd fabricated, from memory.

Civilian life, however, was very different. It felt like I'd lost my military family, the structure, life support and crucially my purpose and meaning. It was almost hero to zero in very quick succession, or so it felt. In addition I missed the adventure, and the variety too. Having left school at 16 I'd known nothing but the Army; I'd never had any other job apart from school-boy and soldier.

I was initially self-employed in 2013 and didn't really know what I was doing. In the military it's all about service and working to achieve the mission, not about making a profit. It was about supporting a team to get the job done, not to fill the coffers of an organisation. In short, I didn't have a clue about making money or a profit or business. As a result, I was burning myself out, working all hours of the day and night to try and gain some traction.

In Christmas 2013 the wheels came off. On Christmas eve my father had gone into hospital for a skin cancer operation and that proved to be a tipping point. My lack of resilience, already low from lack of sleep, opened the door to debilitating anxiety. I began ruminating about the loss of my mother and brother and I was worried that I'd lose the only immediate family I had left – my father. This resulted in me not sleeping for several days. I was extremely wired.

I'd also had heart palpitations and thought I was going to have a heart attack, so ended up sleeping in my van outside A & E at one stage. My slightly skewed logic was that if I had a heart attack outside A & E they wouldn't have far to come and get me. Ultimately and reluctantly I went to my GP for help. My GP prescribed Diazepam sleeping tablets and said that I was probably suffering from Generalised Anxiety Disorder (GAD). In more simple terms, I was mentally and physically knackered and struggling to find my way in an alien world. If any label was appropriate it would probably have been Adjustment Disorder, following on from a stressful life event, namely that of transitioning from soldier to civilian after 24 years of service.

Labels don't always serve us; people talk about 'my depression' or 'my anxiety' as if it's a badge which relinquishes them from any responsibility. Uncomfortable though it may sound, labels can disempower a person. When an individual decides to take responsibility for his or her actions and life strategies, that person can then regain control, take back power too. It's not the GAD that's the issue, it's the way we sometimes think about life and our strategies. They either work for or against us. Perhaps it's the way we bury or suppress our emotions, refuse to dig in and face the problem head-on, or refuse to talk about it and take action too.

My thinking patterns and life strategies were simply not serving me. I was dumping mental and physical fuel at every turn. Having buried, boxed off and suppressed the death of my mother and brother and done very little grieving, it was only a matter of time before it would come back to bite me – like the old adage, *what we resist persists*. Expression, not suppression, is the way ahead.

As a bloke, ex-military too, it can be hard to show emotion and hard to talk about feelings but I'm learning more every day. Every experience we go through in life is valuable. However, the real value isn't truly realised if we don't capture the lessons from such experiences and repurpose them. In the work I do now, I've repurposed my experiences – whether from childhood in Brook Manor, dealing with loss, military training, deployment experience or dealing with transition. It may be tough now but it's in adversity that we often find our new calling, our new purpose and meaning. When I work with clients, either on a one-to-one coaching basis or introducing them to new outdoor experiences and adventure, I've one key aim: to help that person to empower themselves.

Struggle and challenge will always be part of human life. It's how we choose to tackle it, interpret it, and what we choose to do with it, that really counts.

About John

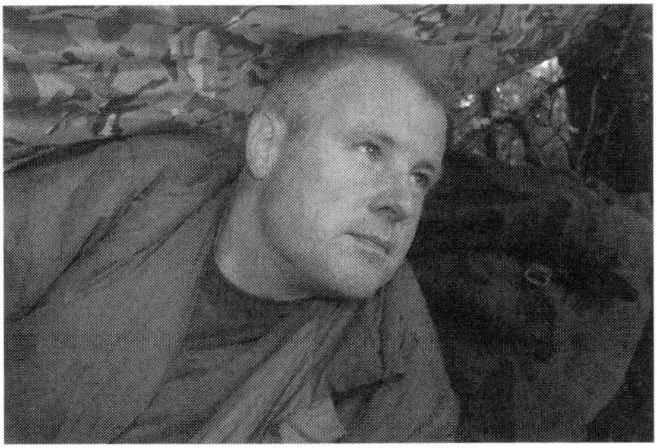

John Watson Allison served with the British Army for 24 years, specialising in Bomb Disposal and Counter-Terrorist Search with the Royal Engineers and latterly Improvised Explosive Device (IED) Intelligence with the Intelligence Corps.

John went on to become a health and wellbeing manager for two London agencies and founded coaching, mentoring and employee wellbeing business, Motion to Mind™ and urban mind/body adventure, StreetGym®. More recently he's launched the *Under a Tarp Challenge* in support of the homeless and to encourage people to learn new, deeply empowering life skills. John is also a Fellow of the Royal Geographical Society, a TEDx speaker, podcaster and author.

Connect with John

www.twitter.com/MotiontoMind

www.twitter.com/TheStreetgym

www.facebook.com/MotionToMind

www.facebook.com/thestreetgym

www.facebook.com//underatarp

www.instagram.com/motion_to_mind

www.instagram.com/streetgym

www.instagram.com/underatarp

www.youtube.com/motiontomind

https://www.youtube.com/motiontomind

www.youtube.com/channel/
UC6_5_1QzdbZbu0fwYnOmw2Q

www.youtube.com/channel/
UC5ZNjQc9Yz28phrb0shQ9jw

enquiries@motiontomind.co.uk

enquiries@streetgym.com

enquiries@underatarp.co.uk

I wish I were dead

Bob Hayward

'Oh, I wish I were dead!' This phrase could be heard many times each day in the corridors of Stone House Hospital. One elderly female patient would punch out this phrase frequently. She was six-feet tall, broad-shouldered, and with unkempt stringy white hair. While well-built for her advanced years, she had been treated with a lobotomy 40 years earlier to cure her of a bipolar disorder. Unfortunately, the lobotomy did not cure this clever, articulate young lawyer. It reduced her to an empty shell. Four decades on she still roamed aimlessly around this large Victorian mental asylum, not knowing what she was saying or doing.

I met her in 1981 on secondment during my psychiatric nurse training. Never did I think I would ever utter that phrase myself, let alone mean it.

In 2017 my life was turned upside down. I was being accused of some horrid things. My integrity and reputation were being questioned; the core of my being was brought down; and everything I stood for was disregarded. Everything I had done for those in need in my local community was trashed and made sordid. A charity I had invested years in supporting was being ripped apart for selfish reasons which could have left those most in need without anywhere to turn to for support.

No smoke without fire, right? The central figure in this dispute was able to create a groundswell of anger against me. For some, the truth is not important. For some, winning while another is destroyed is OK. The ends justify the means. Power corrupts. This fight was, at its heart, a fight for power, a fight between selfless generosity and selfish ambition.

As a Christian, as a happily married man, as a business consultant and as a trustee of a charity I cared deeply about, I could not bring myself to 'fight dirty' as my accuser was. Nor could I bring myself to walk away from the situation. Walking away is not in my nature, no more than stealing from a charity or assaulting another person, sexually or otherwise. I fought and fought and fought – ethically, with the support of my family, and legally, with the support of the other trustees and main financial contributors to the charity. For over a year I fought, with money, time and energy draining me. My business suffered with the turnover down 60%, my income went down, and my costs went up. The charity I was desperately trying to save saw a huge rise in costs, mainly legal costs involved in fighting the attack.

Every day, every waking hour, there was only one thing on my mind: how to stop what I loved, this charity and my own life, being torn down – down, down, down. My mood, my weight, my energy, my finances – down, down, down. The financial reserves at the charity, the resolve of the trustees, the backing of our supporters – down, down, down.

I cannot remember the day when I first said those words to myself: 'I wish I were dead'. I do remember that once said that thought lingered. It became a resident in my mind, a neighbour to every troubled thought, an answer to my biggest fears.

The decision to close the charity and end the fight was taken from me. The trustees and sponsors put the organisation into liquidation. The attacks stopped. The struggle for power ended and so did my reason for existing. That was the worst moment. Never have I felt so defeated, so disjointed, so empty. Never have I rattled around in my head so aimlessly, just like that poor lady all those years before in Stone House. I wished I were dead.

For months afterwards the temptation of suicide was my ever-present silent partner. My family and friends could see I was 'depressed'. I could not hide my low moods and did not have any interest in trying. What little client work I had forced me to put on a front so to the delegates on my leadership or sales training courses I was still the same enthusiastic trainer. That took even more energy from me.

I never told anyone about my silent partner. Walking along the South West Coastal Path one bright sunny day with my wife, Julie, the urge to throw myself over the edge swept over me like the waves rolling in and out of the rocks below. Every few steps the whispering voice called to me again. And again. And again. I stopped and sat silently for some time. Julie knew I was hurting. She sat with me, held my hand, and gave what comfort she could. But without knowing the depth of my despair, without hearing the whispered call to jump and without knowing I was wishing for my life to end – what comfort could she, or anyone give? After a rest, and feeling a little more composed, I asked to call it a day as the heat was getting to me, and so we went back to the hotel.

On 28 August 2018, late in the evening, I was driving back from Bristol Airport when Julie called to say one of my best friends, Carole Ambrose, had died. She had lost her fight with cancer. The urge to undo my seat belt and flip the car over was unbearable. I cried and screamed – at the loss of Carole, at the loss of so many things I held dear. It felt like I had lost my life already. I wished I were dead.

I did not crash the car. You probably worked that out because I am still alive to write these words more than two years afterwards. I did cry and wail for the thirty minutes I took to drive home. That night I fell asleep feeling guilty for not flipping the car over. I felt like a coward, like a cheat. The thought of suicide was becoming more than an impulse; it was becoming a conviction. Not if but when.

What changed?

Julie had encouraged me to go to the Doctor. While he did refer me for talking therapy, he did not take me seriously or show any genuine interest. The talking therapy offered was group-based Cognitive Behavioural Therapy (CBT), just like so many of the CBT groups I assisted with during my time as a psychiatric nurse at Guy's Hospital 40 years before. I could not bring myself to go. OK, I did go to the introductory session but I absolutely hated it. I felt annoyed for the other patients because it was so badly run.

The same week as Carole's death one of my clients was diagnosed with depression, a very intelligent and very able director who had done exceptionally well for his company. Normally he was full of ideas and thought-provoking questions, but now he was morose – barely able to string two words together, unable to do much more than stare aimlessly out of a window.

I was working as a coach to some of the company's managers at this time and was asked by the chief executive to have a session with the director just in case I could help. This meeting forced me to pull out my CBT text books and self-help books from my psychiatric nursing days. I wanted to remind myself of some of the specific questioning techniques because a business coach and a psychotherapist are not the same thing. I also had to remind myself of some of the exercises for the client and which initial programme of client assignments might have the best impact and lift the director's mood.

I bought an Audible version of one of the books so I could listen to it on the way to the director's office. I replayed the initial intervention chapter three times on the drive to meet him that first time. The first session went OK in my mind, and well enough for the director that he agreed to have weekly sessions until he met with his clinical psychologist. I made it clear I was not a CBT specialist and had not practised as a therapist; I was only a sticky plaster, just something better than nothing for a few weeks.

The day after, his boss called me and asked what I had done because the director was 'a changed man' – not his normal self yet, just obviously much better.

I continued to see this director once a week for 60 to 90 minutes each time. I continued to read the CBT books and to revise the next series of questions and exercises on the drive to his office. I also started listening to the CBT book on the drive home from each meeting – to get ahead with my preparation and planning. Seven weeks passed. He had his appointment with his doctor, and we stopped our sessions.

That day, driving home from that last session, I realised something. I realised that my silent partner, my ever-present whispering voice wishing I were dead, was missing. Gone. I smiled to myself, something I had not done for a very long time. Of course, in front of Julie or my children, friends, or clients, I would smile but I did not mean it. I did not smile on the inside and I had not smiled when on my own, not for months – probably over twelve months.

There is plenty of evidence that helping someone else is one of the best ways to help ourselves. There is evidence that our sense of wellbeing can benefit from helping others to regulate their emotions. This can help us regulate our own emotions, lifting our own mood.

While I refused the CBT group therapy, I could not refuse the call to help someone else. While I did not consciously practise the CBT exercises on myself, I was going over and over them so I was familiar enough to explain them to my client – reading, listening and verbalising. This unintended self-help programme driven out of the desire to help another saved my life.

Whether we are the ones providing the emotional support or the ones seeking it, both parties benefit from the display of authentic empathy (acceptance and validation of feelings) and reassessment (applying different perspectives to the situation). By helping others deal with difficult and stressful situations we practise and enhance our own skills at regulating emotions.

At times when the weight of our emotions becomes too much to bear, many of us turn to others for support. For some, the weight of emotions becomes so great that they stop looking for support. That was me. Negative emotions and thought patterns can and do kill.

If you've not yet been (and I pray that you never are) in a place where you can see no other way to relieve the pain other than ending your life, then it is hard to imagine what has led another to commit suicide. There may not always be clear warning signs. Had Julie known or sensed the depth of my despair she would never have agreed to walk along the cliff edge in Cornwall that day or tell me about Carole's death when I was alone driving a car. She did not know. I never said.

It is a myth that the people who do talk about committing suicide never do. Plenty do talk about wanting to die and do take that fateful step. It is important to always take someone seriously if they talk about feeling suicidal. Helping them get the support they need could save their life.

The Samaritans suggest that as many as one in five people has thought about suicide at one time in their life. For most people feeling actively suicidal is temporary. Many people who feel suicidal do not actually want to die; they simply do not want to live the life they have and can see no alternative. I did not really want to kill myself. I just did not want to accept what had happened and did not want to be without the life I once had.

Suicide is often a taboo subject and yet evidence shows that asking someone if they are suicidal can protect them. By asking someone who you know is feeling extremely low about suicide you give them permission to tell you how they feel. People who have felt suicidal will often say what a huge relief it was to be able to talk about what they were experiencing. When we are genuinely listened to we gain attention, acceptance and approval. Listening can be a massive injection of hope and perspective. That injection could be a lifesaver.

If someone does let you know that they are having suicidal thoughts, please take them seriously. You do not have to be able to solve their problems. What you can do is listen and encourage them to talk about how they are feeling. After that you can encourage them to seek help or maybe call The Samaritans (116 123 in the UK).

About Bob

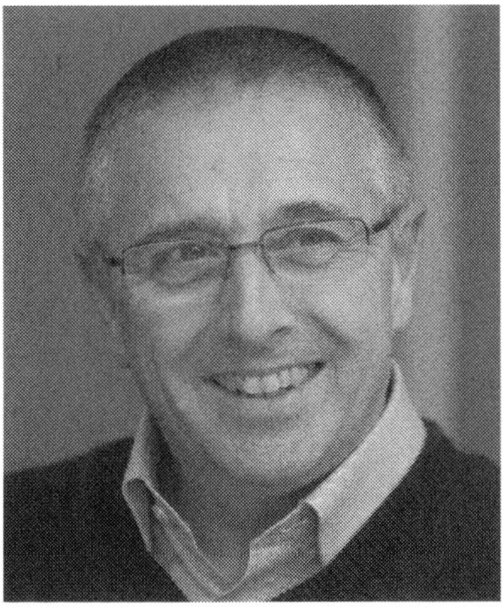

Bob is a Christian, father of four, grandfather of five (so far), Tottenham Hotspur fan and owner of two companies.

He has designed and delivered numerous mission-critical internal communication projects and a huge number of skill development programmes for companies big and small. The author of four bestselling books, he is a highly regarded consultant, trainer and speaker.

An entrepreneur with seven successful start-ups under his belt, he has a wealth of practical experience that makes him a natural and informative speaker with a complete understanding of the needs of employees and the problems facing business owners and managers.

Bob has previously co-authored four Amazon bestsellers:

Persuade: How to persuade anyone about anything

Remote Working: How to effectively and efficiently work from home in challenging times

Fit for Purpose Leadership #6

Pivot & Grow

And the most recent *The Profit Secret.*

Connect with Bob

www.bemoreeffective.com

www.linkedin.com/in/bobhayward

www.twitter.com/bobhayward

The Mask

Raj Koria

'How are you?'

'I'm fine.'

If I'd had enough to drink, I wouldn't feel the constriction in my chest that occurred whenever I gave that answer. It was that tell-tale sign that I wasn't being honest; that reminder that I wasn't actually fine; that things were going on behind the facade of my smile that were causing me anxiety, keeping me up at night, and really making me struggle and despair at times. But I could never tell anyone this – whether it was friends, family, or even my wife at the time. I could not risk letting anyone know that things were not fine. I wouldn't dare let the mask slip.

I was never taught how to handle emotions, especially negative ones. Even as a child, crying was not an acceptable reaction to anything. I was taught how to 'do' – study hard, work hard, be respectable. But I didn't know how to feel. So when things were difficult, I got on with it (or at least I tried to). I was 21 when my dad died. My brother came with a car full of uncles and cousins to break the news to me. As soon as I saw them pull up, I knew what had happened and I started crying where I stood. One of my cousins remarked, 'I thought you were strong', the implication being that by crying I was being weak. It worked. I stopped crying. I pretended to be 'strong' which meant bottling up my emotions and letting them fester inside me. I don't blame my cousin. He hadn't been taught to deal with negative emotions either, so my crying made him uncomfortable and he wanted me to stop. I was the same.

Throughout my life, whenever anyone asked me how I was, I protected them from the difficulty of dealing with my emotions by pretending that I was fine. In most cases we were both colluding in the lie. I didn't want to tell them how I actually was and, in most cases, they didn't really want to know. Like my cousin, it would most likely have been uncomfortable for them, were I to answer truthfully. So we had an unwritten social contract where they would ask the question and I would give the answer they wanted to hear. And vice versa.

What did I get out of it? How did it benefit me to hide myself away like that? Looking back I realise I was motivated by a fear of being rejected. I was convinced that people didn't want to know about my emotions, my 'weaknesses'. It was far easier for them to know that I was happy and well; that I was fine. If I went around breaking that social contract, they wouldn't want to know me; they would reject me. I wanted to be socially accepted and so, to achieve that, I played by what I thought were the rules.

Yet the cost to me of doing this was immense. I was never truly close to anyone – not my family, not my best friends, not my girlfriends and not my ex-wife. The reason for this was they only saw the mask. They only saw the person who was 'fine'. They never saw the real me, warts and all. They never saw the sadness, the tears, the fears, the self doubts. Sure, some of those things no doubt came across in my behaviour, but I never expressed them. So, if I was unable to express fundamental truths about myself even to those I was closest to, it shouldn't really be a surprise that there was always a barrier between us and those relationships never grew deeper beyond a certain point.

One casualty of this was my marriage. I cannot pinpoint when things started to go wrong in that relationship but by the time one of us finally plucked up the courage to openly admit to the other that things were not well (no prizes for guessing that it wasn't me who took this step), it was too late and the relationship was beyond repair. In reality it was clear that things had been going badly for at least a couple of years but throughout that time I did not speak to anyone about it. I pretended everything was fine. Even when my ex-wife finally spoke up about it, rather than open up, express my emotions and explain what was going on with me, I resolved to 'try harder' and made sure that mask was securely on. A month later the relationship was over. Other relationships came and went, suffering a similar fate.

Perhaps the biggest impact of this constant masking over my true self was on my well-being. Not being able to be genuinely close to anyone meant that I was fundamentally lonely throughout a lot of my life. I felt isolated from others. Only now can I see the irony of this, considering one of the reasons I hid my feelings was that I didn't want to be rejected. Over time this took its toll on my mental health, in particular in the form of addictive behaviours, which were fuelled by loneliness and isolation. Even as things got worse for me, I continued to be 'fine' whenever asked, holding onto that mask ever tighter, thus prolonging that sense of loneliness and isolation which in turn made me feel worse. It was a long, slow, downward spiral.

It is only now I have begun to change these patterns in my life that I am able to look back and see what they were and what impact they had. More importantly, I am able to see the benefits of doing things differently.

So what was it that got me to change and take off that mask of being fine? I cannot identify one single action that brought about the change but I got to a point in my life where the loneliness and isolation I felt outweighed the fear of showing my real self and being rejected.

I had moved back to London after living abroad. It was a little while after I got divorced and I was looking forward to reconnecting with all my many friends in London after being away for eight years. I thought I would have a ready-made social network which would mean I could avoid feeling alone. Except it didn't work out that way. Most of my friends lived very different lives now and I found that reconnecting with them didn't really happen and, as a result, I had to deal with my loneliness for the first time. In response to this, I decided to make the most of London and get out to meet people. Many people – most – were like me: they wore the mask. But I met some who didn't.

When I asked these people how they were, they gave me an honest answer and I found it a revelation. I connected with them more. Moreover, when they asked me how I was and I responded that I was fine, they saw through it and, in an inquisitive yet caring way, questioned my assertion. When I opened up about myself, they did not reject me, as I always feared would happen. Slowly but surely, I felt safer being honest and revealing my real self. I began to shed the mask.

Now, when asked how I am, before I answer I try to check in with myself and first ask myself the same question. Then I try to give an honest answer, which is not easy. My first instinct is usually still to don that mask of being fine and there are times when I still follow that old pattern. But more often than not I am able to move past that instinct to show some vulnerability and share that I am not necessarily fine. It almost always feels risky doing this, even now. What if it puts them off to have this 'weak' man in front of them? What if they don't want to know me because of that? But that hardly ever happens. Most of the time such openness is met with cautious yet pleasant surprise and it creates a stronger connection with that person by allowing them to get closer to me. They are seeing the real me and they see that I trust them. This, in turn, gives them permission to be honest about themselves too, so more often than not they reciprocate and the connection grows. I suppose you can say that I am paying it forward from those people who did the same for me.

This simple act of being honest about my feelings has helped transform my relationships. I am far closer to friends and to family. My being open and honest has given them 'permission' to open up. We share more about ourselves with each other, about our hopes and dreams as well as our fears and anxieties. Don't get me wrong, there are still conversations about the weather and football but we now also connect on deeper matters and I feel like I know them far better now. This isn't the case with every friend or family member – some have been more receptive to it than others – but I calibrate my responses according to what each person is realistically comfortable with and I keep trying.

My relationship with my girlfriend is unlike any previous relationship I've had. It is open and communicative. I used to have a belief that as a man I needed to show that I was strong in order to be attractive and I could not be strong if I was showing weaknesses, namely my fears and anxieties. But I have learned that this is not true. I can be strong and vulnerable at the same time. In fact, being able to be open and honest about my feelings and about how I am is a sign of strength and self-assuredness. Whereas the inherent dishonesty of the mask of being fine is the opposite; it is a sign of insecurity. So, by being more open about my feelings I have shed a layer of insecurity. Now that I am more honest and far less insecure, I am more connected to my girlfriend than I have been in any relationship.

I have seen changes in my mental health too. Being more connected to people has meant that I feel less lonely and isolated. Constantly hiding who I am and living behind the mask of being fine carried with it a sense of anxiety, anxiety about the mask slipping and the consequences of people finding out what I am really like. Shedding that anxiety has also had a positive affect on me. And this has only been the start. That one change of behaviour – shedding the mask and being honest about myself – and the impact that has had, has started me down a path of really looking after my mental health, of working to improve my understanding of myself and of others. I now use tools like writing out resentments, releasing stuck emotions, journaling about my thoughts and feelings, regularly expressing my fears to friends and confidants, writing out a gratitude list, and many others to help my sense of wellbeing. I deal with my emotions in a way that embraces them as opposed to masking them over. As a result I feel lighter, happier and more comfortable in my own skin. I feel I am more accepted by those around me (ironically) and I feel like I am having a positive impact on their lives which helps me to feel better about myself too.

That one act of shedding the mask of being fine was a difficult thing to get started but the snowballing impact of it in my life has been miraculous.

About Raj

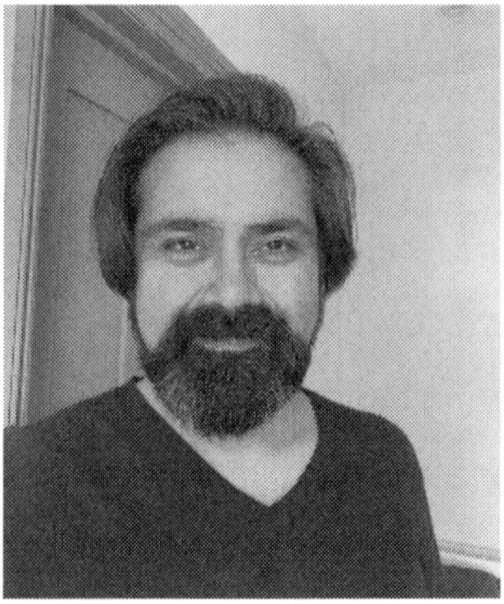

Raj Koria is an international sports lawyer specialising in commercial rights. He runs a sports and media consultancy called Fortus. He lives in London for now but will soon be moving out closer to the countryside so his pet cat, Sky, has a garden to stalk around in.

His loves include cooking, cinema, the National Portrait Gallery and pub quizzes. And Sky, of course.

Connect with Raj

www.instagram.com/RajKoriaLondon

www.twitter.com/The_British_Raj

His Menopause

Mike Sheridan

I didn't know what anxiety was until it became a critical issue for me. I suppose I am from the generation who had no ability to recognise it in all of its forms as we do today. I knew why I was struggling at the time and why I first began to think about self-harming but I was unable to help myself. My first wife and long-term partner had walked out of the family home leaving me, her husband of 17 years, and our daughter.

I know now that suffering from anxiety means we often seek ways to make it stop; the pain is simply too much to carry. I began to look for immediate solutions – once, when walking the dog in some woods and later at home … wherever looked feasible. Initially I just thought about where and how. Then one day I acted things out, making decisions. I wasn't scared, just in a state of constant agony. Physically I was in bad shape too. There was a period when I had not slept for over a week. I'd lost over a stone in weight even though I was eating healthily sometimes, but mostly not. My mind would ruminate over the past in a never-ending loop. I was not living in the present, facing up to reality. I couldn't see a future. Alcohol was a short-term useful release, but I was abusing the distraction far too much.

The cumulative effects built up, adding to my already depressed state. Emotionally and physically I shut down. I became severely impotent which was a shock. There was no life down there whatsoever. I had digestion issues and extreme levels of constipation. As a further consequence my painful anal fissure, or tear, was examined by a doctor. He told me that if ointments didn't help the problem might require surgery.

I could function at my work in corporate sales by turning up, but I was numb in every respect, just existing. My job often involved foreign travel, so I had to plan duties carefully to fit in with my daughter's time with me. With the help of a solicitor I managed to legally secure 50/50 shared care for her. This meant she could spend one week with me and one week with her Mum. There was a time when arrangements had to be enforced because they were not being adhered to. These times were extremely hard on everyone.

To start with I simply couldn't be alone; separation was excruciating. I went to Relate and they stressed the importance of family – which was ironic! What they meant was that I needed to put my lifeboat to sea and choose who I wanted to be in it with me. You know you are in a bad place when relatives make sure you have their number to call day or night.

My lowest point came when I realised I needed to tell someone about my very urgent need to stop my pain. I told my doctor who referred me to a mental health consultant. He also said something I later realised was profoundly helpful: 'Let's get you sleeping first'. The sleeping pills put me under at night but couldn't provide deep sleep. Within a few days I filled in the doctor's forms for a mental health assessment. The consultant only had to ask me what was going on in my life before my tears began to flow. I sat slumped in a chair opposite her blubbering like a child, holding my head in my hands and pleading for help. The mild release was there, like opening a tap to alleviate pressure, but the reservoir of hurt was deep and wide. I was given leaflets about the Samaritans, counselling sessions and cognitive therapy. The consultant reminded me of my responsibility as a father; she was quite firm with me but only after she had witnessed my relief at being able to share my pain. I'd been given the opportunity to talk but also received a talking-to.

I can only describe what followed as a long path towards an inward focus and giving myself some space for healing. I took control of my situation, petitioned for divorce and organised complete financial separation. I was lucky that I had building blocks to make that happen. I'd searched for a lawyer through my network of friends and family, settling on one who showed me how to stay out of the courts. She explained how I could go for a 'clean break', using refinance to keep my home for myself and my daughter as long as we needed it, and how to protect my pension. As my ex was working, and because of shared parenting arrangements, there would be no maintenance required.

At the end of the day courts no longer care who earns the most money, who did the most parenting or who said what to whom. They only intervene if children are in danger of neglect or if the threat of violence exists within the former marital home. It took over a year to finalise everything.

In the years that followed I hunkered down and started to seek healthier distraction therapy for myself than the ones I'd been using. During weekends on my own I swam early, rode my bicycle for miles, exploring new places, cooked healthier meals and went to bed early. I holidayed on my own, driving to remote parts of the country with my bike on the car rack. I went for long walks in the countryside, accompanied by flasks of tea and packed lunches. I chatted with strangers. I started to look forward to quiet early mornings when I could sit in peace and just listen. I decided that the basic truths of life are constantly being transmitted to us but unfortunately unless we orientate ourselves more towards them, we cannot hear them.

Eventually, by taking pleasure in the smaller, free things in life I found a new gratitude for them. I looked forward to solitude without loneliness. When my daughter was with me we did fun things together. I tried to show her that she didn't always have to be busy, doing and achieving. I began to write about my experiences, as a way of processing everything. Initially I thought I was writing about the pain of separation and how I felt there was little help available for men. I posted on blogs about divorce and thought my journey through my struggles had been all about that.

Because I was spending so much time listening for truths, however, something else happened: I developed an understanding of human suffering as an essential part of life. No one is free from it and it moulds who we become. I learnt that the mind and body are not separate.

Relief from emotional pain began for me when I sought to quieten my mind and set aside time for striving to achieve that with daily practice. With my new special friend – time – I began to understand that my daughter's mother had struggled immensely through early menopause. I learnt how hormones are extremely powerful and how chemically manufactured hormones delivered to women via their doctor can have a profound derailing effect on their lives. There is more documentation available now about the physical side effects and potential risks of Hormone Replacement Therapy (HRT) but I could find nothing about the psychological effects. I have spoken to some women who told me that they had to stop taking it because it made them feel 'out of it'. It's known that with certain hormones diminishing naturally, our wives or partners can lose their mothering, nurturing instincts, become less interested in sex, suffer mood swings and be more susceptible to depression. If women are just beginning to understand why and how these things happen during menopause, what chance do men have?!

For me, I likened the experience of being on the receiving end of menopause as living with anything from unpredictable mild premenstrual tension to a constant outpouring of emotion and fits of anger, followed by a steep decline. When people explain – in the really rough seas of life – that everything happens for a reason, in the midst of our own pain the message never lands with us. We are simply not ready or open enough to understand.

I couldn't see the truth of what was happening to my life because I had no reference point. I had also endured many false accusations which I'd believed too readily. Our partners know our weak spots and where to hurt us. I also feel strongly that if women take the pill for many years to prevent conception, followed by drugs to kickstart fertilisation and then HRT to try to mimic the hormone balances of youth, the net result is a series of massive intrusions in the body's intended natural cycles. With HRT, it was a lady doctor who told me: 'the experiment continues'. I was shocked by her honesty. If the pharmaceutical industry is culpable I believe it wouldn't be the first time.

Today I'm pleased to say that I know much more about my own anxiety, and how to continue to work on myself and some of the triggers I need to avoid. My life got better each time I let go of another piece of emotional baggage. I pay attention to how I'm feeling physically, I'm eating cleaner and getting more sleep. I've left the corporate world of unachievable goals and relentless competition. Yes, I ride a bike! I try not to think of myself as a middle-aged man in lycra. I do it because it feels like meditation, boosts my mood and keeps my weight in check. The more I read about its benefits the more I want to ride even if it's just to feel the wind and witness an early morning. I also know that it provides one small element of the adventure missing in many men's lives today which is why so many struggle.

The hunter-gatherer in me understands I need to find the company of other men to share exciting adventures with, not to compete with. I'd like to challenge the notion that men don't talk. Perhaps we don't talk as much as women, but I believe that's by design! *Being fine* for me means I need to be much more aware of how I'm feeling, rejecting negative thoughts. I also need to continue to work on my nutrition, health and fitness and to always, always give myself a break if I slip up mentally. There is a personal responsibility required to get our shit together, accepting at the same time that everyone on the planet is just another soul at their own stage of development. We are all a work in progress and being kinder to ourselves is the key.

About Mike

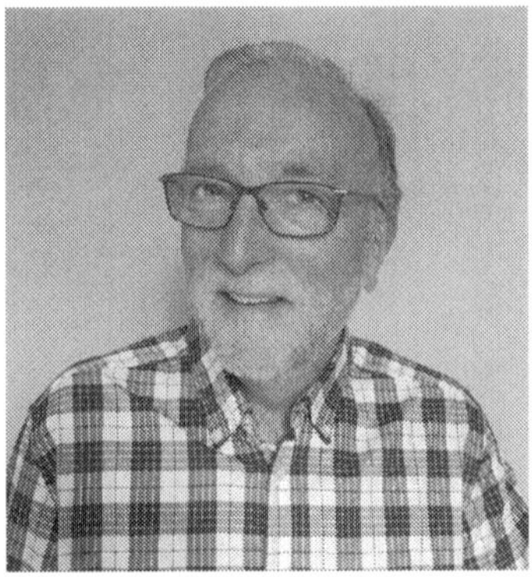

Mike has lived in Ealing, West London for over twenty years. He has worked in the fast-moving world of technology sales since the late 1980s but more recently has stepped out of the hamster wheel to spend more time riding his bike! By finding the space to focus on his personal health and wellbeing he has been rediscovering himself and his priorities.

Mike was married for 17 years to his first wife before petitioning for divorce in 2009. The pain of separation and related circumstances took Mike to the brink. He sought help at his lowest point from his doctor and didn't hold back about how bad he was feeling.

His daughter Jess now lives in Edinburgh, having recently graduated from University. In September 2018 Mike married Claire, having found love again, and Jess was Mike's best man! Mike and Claire have decided to sell up, move out to the West Country and hope to find a new home near the sea.

Connect with Mike

msherihome@aol.com

www.linkedin.com/in/mikesheridandata

The Question a Man Must Always Ask

Laurelle Rond

In today's society many women are at last being freed from the bonds of gender discrimination. Stories of the emotional, physical and sexual abuse they have suffered fill the media channels along with the names of men who are being shamed for the power games they have enacted.

Yet the images of men portrayed through television, films and novels have hardly changed. Attractive, powerful men who are strong, brave heroes still dominate our screens, telling men how they should be if they are to become a 'real' man.

So, what is a 'real' man? Is he the 'Milk Tray' man, that heroic and handsome adventurer who will stop at no physical limits to bring a gift of chocolates to the woman he admires without ever actually touching or even seeing her? Or is he the man who can survive in any environment because he is tough and has no emotional needs whatsoever? Or is he the weeping footballer who drenches the shoulders of anyone who will listen to his dramatic portrayals of all the wrongs that have been done to him?

What it means to be a man today is becoming increasingly fractured, so it is no surprise that boys no longer know who or what they should model themselves on. One story tells them they should be detached, rough heroes whilst another tells them they should be sensitive, caring and gentle. In the end, they must surely be forgiven if they no longer know which way to turn and feel like fools.

We think that this is a modern problem but it has actually existed for centuries. In the 12th century, a writer of French romance, Chrétien de Troyes, wrote the story of Parsifal, describing how a man can learn to become a man whilst also healing his inner Wounded Male. Note the word *inner*. What we have still refused to acknowledge, eight centuries later, is that human life is a balance between inner and outer experience. Male, female or other, we still seek to focus our attention on our outer experience and ignore the inner work which needs to be done if any form of sustainable peace or happiness is ever to be attained.

The story of Parsifal is the story of how a boy becomes a man and all the obstacles that he must face if he is to become his real self. It goes something like this:

Once upon a time, there was a castle. In this castle was the Holy Grail. The King of the Grail Castle was the Fisher King but he had been so grievously wounded in his genitals that he couldn't live nor could he die and his suffering caused desolation amongst his people and the land.

Meanwhile, a boy was born in Wales who was so insignificant and uneducated that he didn't even have a name. He was raised by his mother alone because his father and brothers had all been killed.

One day, when he was a young teenager, the boy saw five knights riding by. He was so dazzled that he rushed home to tell his mother, pleading with her to let him join them. Heartbroken, his mother nevertheless gave him her blessing. But before he left, she instructed him to respect fair damsels, not to ask too many questions and to wear a homespun garment that she had woven to keep him warm.

Once the boy had set off on his quest to become a knight, he was told to make his way to King Arthur's court. But when he arrived, he was laughed at by everyone, not least by a humourless damsel who hadn't smiled for six years. This gave the boy his name – Parsifal – which means Innocent Fool.

There are many quests in this long story as Parsifal goes on to slay dragons, conquer knights and rescue fair maidens but it is not until he receives three more instructions that he finally discovers just how to become one of Arthur's Knights – the apparent pinnacle of all-male achievement. The instructions are that he must never seduce or be seduced by a fair maiden; he must find the Grail Castle and the Fisher King, and ask 'Whom does the Grail Serve?'

After he has discovered that his beloved mother has died of a broken heart, he falls in love with the damsel he has rescued – Blanche Fleur – but refuses to consummate the relationship. After that he finds the Grail Castle and the Fisher King but, because his mother had told him not to ask too many questions, he fails to ask 'Whom does the Grail serve?' And because of this the Fisher King, who represents the Wounded Masculine, is not healed and Parsifal is forced to continue searching for his knighthood.

So far, not so good.

It isn't until he becomes overcome with love for the seemingly unattainable Blanche Fleur that he once more returns to the Castle where he is given his second opportunity to ask the all-important question. But again he remains silent. As a result he is forced to listen to a long and humiliating list of all his failures which nearly brings him to his knees. It is only when he finds himself in front of the Fisher King for the third time that he at last dares to ask the all-important question – 'Whom Does the Grail Serve?'

As if by magic, the Fisher King is instantly healed and able to drink from the Grail. Immediately the crops and animals grow strong as do the hearts and happiness of all his people. Best of all, Parsifal is finally able to become one of Arthur's legendary Knights of the Round Table.

This tale of quests and rescues, sieges and battles, shows us how a man earns his manhood in stages from his devotion to his mother, to being forced to listen to the humiliating list of his failures, to his inability to have a real relationship with a woman, to his refusal to ask that most vital of questions – 'Whom does the Grail Serve?' ... to his eventual understanding that nothing will be achieved if he does not ask that question.

The question seems to be the point of the story but what does it actually mean?

As well as sharing this story Chrétien de Troyes, conceived of a dish large enough to hold a salmon – a Celtic symbol of wisdom. Unfortunately, de Troyes died before he actually revealed the origin of the Grail. Nevertheless, other writers, including Dan Brown, soon began to take up the story and the most common explanation has become that the Holy Grail was the cup that Christ drank from at the Last Supper, another symbol of spiritual wisdom.

And so we begin to understand that Parsifal has to learn wisdom before he can earn his place at Arthur's Round Table. If we think of the Grail as a chalice, it is not unlike a cauldron which is a symbolic container of the Feminine. And here we arrive at the crux of the matter. We human beings are deeply divided in ourselves – a division represented by the Masculine and Feminine. Our spiritual purpose is to bring together the separated halves of ourselves in a Divine Marriage.

Carl Jung suggested that a man would only ever achieve his manhood when he connected with the female inside himself – his *anima* – just as a woman would only ever achieve her full potential when she connected with the male inside herself – her *animus*. Parsifal's ultimate quest, therefore, is his inner work – the uniting of the two halves of himself – and to do this he must engage with his *anima* and enable the Divine Marriage of Masculine and Feminine within.

To understand this internal journey, let's look at the archetypes of the *anima* and *animus*. Archetypal traits are divided into light and shadow: the light qualities are the ones we will happily own, whereas the shadow qualities are those we refuse to acknowledge and therefore project onto others.

Parsifal's external, swashbuckling quests develop the light qualities of his Divine Masculine – the *animus*, for example: assertiveness, courage, analytical thought, strength, vitality, decisiveness, a focused attentiveness and a desire for achievement. In order to develop his potential, however, and discover who he really is inside, he must develop his *anima* – his Divine Feminine – and it is for this purpose that he must ask the question, 'Whom Does the Grail Serve?' The meaning of this question now starts to become clear. If developing our opposite side leads us to develop our spirituality, then this is the Grail that we are seeking.

For Parsifal, the Grail serves his Divine Feminine. By asking the question he unites his *animus* and *anima* and the wounded Fisher King is healed. This means that Parsifal will now acknowledge the archetypes of his *anima* – such as feelings, emotions, tenderness, relatedness, commitment and fidelity, friendship, love and compassion, imagination, gentleness, romance, creativity, intuition and a sense of aesthetics.

Parsifal misses the first two opportunities to ask the question because he is not yet old or mature enough to have sufficient confidence and wisdom to dare to embrace his female qualities as well as the masculine qualities that he is actively seeking. Because he is still abiding by other people's instructions, he is also not yet ready to heal the Divine Masculine as represented by the Fisher King.

The Fisher King is a tragic character; loved by his people, his suffering makes everything and everyone desolate. This is what men are facing today. When there is no place for the archetypal Masculine side to develop naturally, then a man is unable to find out who he truly is. He yearns to develop only the light qualities in himself but how can he do this when being a knight is impossible in today's culture? And if he can't develop his masculinity in a safe, acceptable way then how on earth is he going to be able to develop his *anima* which will require him to become vulnerable – a frightening and shocking state of mind feared by most men.

If vulnerability frightens someone, it will take them in one of two directions: the shadow Feminine – in other words moodiness, sentimentality, hysteria, possessiveness and withdrawal; or the shadow Masculine – in other words aggression, ruthlessness, argumentativeness and mechanistic behaviour. When a man finds his Inner Female threatening, he is likely to do everything he can to avoid developing his *anima*. This is why a father might seek to break his daughter's spirit in an attempt to reduce her to less than himself. This is why a brother might try to control his sisters in case they show him up to be less than he should be. This is why a husband might do everything he can to make his wife small enough to fit in with his warped, tiny and distorted vision of himself.

The Divine Feminine – *anima* – in Parsifal's life is represented by several characters. Amongst these is his mother who holds onto him for too long by exhorting him not to ask too many questions and by insisting that he wear her homespun. He should have taken the garment off when he won the Red Knight's armour but instead he tries to force this new garment over the top of the old. This causes him to be ridiculed again and further undermines his masculinity, as represented by the serious damsel who laughs when she sees the naïve, nameless boy.

But because this is one of the stages that he must go through, he at last earns his name – remember that Parsifal means The Innocent Fool. His Divine Feminine is then represented by Blanche Fleur, a damsel he has rescued from a siege. However, he is so determined to stick to the instructions he has been given that he refuses to consummate the relationship and instead only gives her a chaste kiss. This is symbolic of him seeing his *anima* but refusing to fully engage with it.

Another, rather brutal symbol of his *anima* is the Hideous Damsel who regales him with all of his failures, but then the Old Hermit does the same so it seems that humiliation is the prerogative in the development of both *anima* and *animus*.

In the end, irrespective of gender, human life is all about learning how to make ourselves whole. Experience tends to fragment us over and over again until we can learn how to sew ourselves back up again and regain our centre. Parsifal shows us just how painful this can be and also that we will fail many times before we finally succeed. Just as women are coming out of their shells and discovering how much they can *do* by developing their *animus*, men are also being challenged to discover all that they can *be* by developing their *anima*.

Parsifal's quests are necessary because they are full of action and decisiveness, focus and clarity, strength and courage. But until he discovers his feminine side and dares to touch Blanche Fleur properly instead of keeping her at a chaste arm's length, he will never unite the two parts of himself that cannot, ultimately, live without each other. He is looking for his Other Half and, until he finds that part of himself, like the Fisher King, he will not be healed.

A healed man loves completely and honestly both internally and externally. He combines strength with vulnerability, courage with compassion and focus with creativity. This is not about gender – there are all sorts of genders amongst humanity – but about the divisions of the soul being healed. Only by integrating himself into a whole will he be able to hold his humanity in his hands with a heart, mind and spirit as big as the world he lives in. Only by loving his beloved in a real, human way will his knighthood and compassionate selves unite.

And only by asking the Grail question, and receiving the answer, will he be sufficiently healed to achieve his ambition of joining King Arthur's Round Table – round because it symbolises the infinite spirit that is wise in all things and never-ending.

Once he does this, he will at last become a true knight, a glorious creature and beacon of light to all boys, youths and men who follow him.

As long as they, of course, also – in their turn – ask the question...

About Laurelle

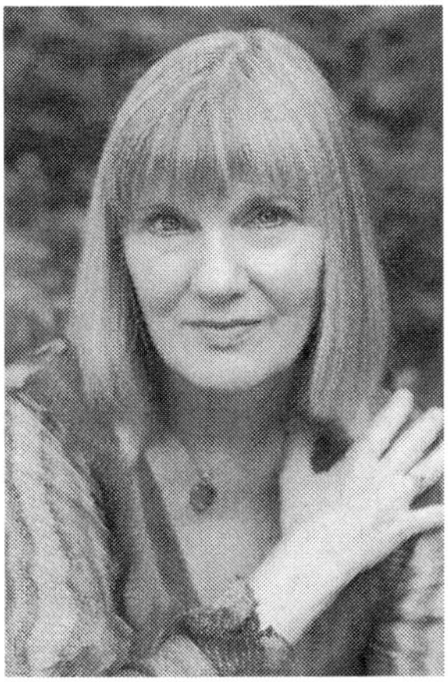

Laurelle Rond began her career as a musician, singer and writer. By combining all these elements she has developed a method of healing using therapeutic sound and is a qualified and experienced Sound Therapist.

Laurelle became interested in Greek mythology when a study of archetypes led her to research the role of healing in human psychology. As a result, she now runs workshops on spiritual and psychological development as well as working extensively with the voice as a practical method of empowerment.

Her first novel was published in 2012 and she has just finished her third. She has also recorded 12 CDs.

Connect with Laurelle

www.laurellerond.com

www.conscious-tuning.com/

www.facebook.com/LaurelleRondSound

www.linkedin.com/in/yoursound

www.twitter.com/LaurelleRond

The Old Me, Depressed Me & New Me

Steve McDermott

'In the depth of winter, I finally learned that there was in me an invincible summer.'

Albert Camus

Prologue

When I was extremely unwell with clinical depression there is no way I could have read a whole book, never mind just one chapter, on why – particularly as a man – I needed to talk to someone. I was far too ashamed, mentally and physically exhausted and lacking any form of concentration. Even if I'd found the energy needed that I was always sadly lacking, I would not have believed one bloody word that told me I could recover – ever. I was convinced I was broken and could never be fixed. If you are currently suffering you might well believe the same thing. Put this book down if you want; it will still be there when the time is right. Or give it to a loved one, friend or colleague so they might get a better understanding of this illness. Most of all it will help comfort them and will help them hold on to the hope and belief that you will get better, even if you don't believe that yourself just yet.

Act 1: The Old Me

Listen, I'm from Yorkshire and around these parts we're not fond of big heads. However, it's important you know a bit about the old me to understand how I ended up in the new place I now find myself.

From when I was a kid, I've always been a great talker, and creative and an extrovert by nature. So it should come as no surprise that I enjoyed a very successful 15-year career as Creative Director of an advertising agency. During my time in advertising we were the documentary version of the TV series Madmen; the ability to generate wild ideas, demonstrate extreme self-confidence and drink lots of champagne were prerequisites.

Then, in a wild career switch, having discovered the power of personal development, I started my own company to help others become more confident and successful.

From there I was headhunted by an agent and my life and work went international when I became a professional motivational speaker. My style of straight-talking with an element of stand-up comedy proved very popular to thousands of people all around the world. I won The European Motivational Speaker of the Year award three times. I wrote an international bestselling book, using my trademark Yorkshire sense of humour, that helped loads of people lead more happy, successful and fulfilled lives.

Audience members have described me as: 'like a tornado through a caravan park'; 'a one-man whirlwind'; and 'more energy than the Duracell Bunny!'

You could say I was, without doubt, much more than a glass half-full type of person. In fact, I was a glass full to the brim of optimism, positive ideas, emotions and actions. It was my purpose as a performer to inspire others and bring that love of life and success to the masses.

Not only had I been happily married for over 25 years to the marvellous Candy and with three equally wonderful grown-up children, I also had all the material stuff other people often associate with happiness.

What could possibly go wrong?

Act 2: The Depressed Me

There are times when we are feeling down in the dumps, having a bad day or temporarily in a low mood. We all have those – unless you are one of those annoyingly, relentlessly positive types. However, don't tell someone to 'Just cheer up mate' when that person may be suffering from a disease of the mind. Thing is, you might not know you are mentally unwell unless you've been properly diagnosed. If you're not sure, the first port of call should be your doctor, hopefully a good one.

Did I just wake up one day a bit sad? No. Nor am I going to describe in vivid detail my almost imperceptible decline from the happy-go-lucky me to the non-functioning shell of a man who would google 'best ways to kill yourself' not because I wanted to die but because I just wanted the pain to end.

I know you are really curious as to what caused my mental ill health. People always are. It's the first question they always ask – just like my doctor did – especially when you tell them your job is a motivational speaker!

Here's the thing … whether it's brain chemistry, inflammation, life events, an accident or something else entirely, science can't seem to agree on what causes depression. For all I know it could be a mixture of them all! If you're not careful, you'll spend far too much time discussing and analysing what caused your depression. We never figured out exactly what caused mine. I fell down the stairs and broke my ribs; maybe that was the start. Who knows? I had severe clinical depression, twice.

If we had known the causes, don't you think we would have solved it dead quickly? It might be a good idea not to tell certain people in order to avoid endless repetitions of the 'Umm, I wonder what caused it?' type of conversation. Because they care, people – especially men – often want to find quick solutions to your problems. I much prefer Candy's approach. She says: 'Sometimes depression just IS.'

However, if I'd not pretended to be fine for so long, I do wonder if it would have saved me at least two wasted years of my life – often spent mainly in bed, on my own, in the dark, in torment (turns out they were not wasted but I was yet to realise that).

If you've already read some of the other chapters in this book you will understand that mental ill health is a unique experience for everyone.

What I can say is that generally depression is massively misunderstood – ironically, most often (just like yours truly) by the sufferers themselves. You see I used to believe that there must be a clear reason why you got depressed and that you had a choice if it happened to you or not. I naively thought some people were mentally tough and others were not.

One of our daily newspapers has a feature where they ask celebrities about their health. You know, questions like: 'Can you still run up a flight of stairs?' They also ask, 'Have you ever suffered from depression?' Most of the replies are words to the effect of: 'Well I've always been a glass half-full type of person,' or 'Mentally I'm very strong'. The biggest misunderstanding of all regarding depression is that not just celebrities but also the vast majority of the population believe that there's some form of choice involved.

What I now know is that depression is a non-discriminatory, equal opportunities disease. It could infect as many as one in four people, possibly more in the times we now live in. This misunderstanding is often why the ill person can feel so ashamed because they wrongly believe they are weak and just need to 'Man up'. And why is there sadly still such a big stigma attached to any form of mental illness? You need to know it can happen to anyone at any time.

I'm happy to tell anyone, especially men, that I've had mental health challenges in the past. I felt it should no longer be kept a secret or something to be ashamed of. It had ceased to be so misunderstood and surely things have moved on since I first confessed[2] to having depression several years ago. Turns out I was wrong – hence the need for a book like this.

Why is that?

When I was growing up, we were taught that men don't show vulnerabilities. The belief that 'you must never show weakness' was deeply ingrained in me from a young age.

My grandad fought in the first world war and was shot through both legs on the first day of the Battle of the Somme. After the war, he was a miner working in the tough conditions of the county Durham coalfields. Then he was thrown out of work for leading the miners out on strike. I never really knew or saw him. I have just one vivid memory as a small boy of visiting him when he was elderly at what I've since discovered was High Royds Psychiatric Hospital, just before he died. At the time it felt like he was some kind of secret and was being hidden away. Today I can make an educated guess as to why he was there.

Simply put, I learnt from an early age that boys don't cry. Does this traditional view of manhood still exist? In a recent study of young men in Mexico, the UK and the USA, researchers identified a set of beliefs that

2. *As a lapsed Catholic, the word 'confess' strikes me as interesting in relation to mental health 'issues'. As does 'issues'. I wonder if anyone would ever have to 'confess' to having issues with cancer or a broken leg? People still say to me things like: 'Of all the people I know, I never thought you were the type to get depression.' We have a long way to go before things change.*

place pressure on men to behave in a certain way. The researchers concluded that these pressures tell men to be self-sufficient and act tough. They were trapped within a set of socially reinforced rules about what 'real men' should do, a version of manhood that has no place for the vulnerable.

Can you now see why in the depths of my depression – like when I burst into floods of tears over something as trivial as the cat being sick on the carpet – I wasn't about to rush off and tell anyone about it? I wasn't going to tell anyone why I felt less of a man and why I was ashamed.

To overcome the myth of what it means to be a 'real man' is hard. We're not great at talking about our feelings even when we are healthy! At first it was near impossible to talk about how I actually felt. I'd go further and say all the well-meaning campaigns that tell us 'It's good to talk' miss the point. Most people just can't find the words. I simply couldn't articulate what was going on inside my head – those dark thoughts – or begin to convey my despair and pain, and I'm a professional speaker! A foggy brain and faulty thinking didn't help.

My wife's endless patience, non-judgemental attitude and willingness to just listen or, in my case, read what I had to say without offering solutions, did help. Always remember there is a big difference between telling people you are depressed and being able to actually talk about it.

Eventually, I got up enough courage to tell a few other people apart from close family and friends. And do you know what? It was such a relief because the energy needed to put on a brave face and keep up appearances is draining.

You will also be amazed how many other people are going through or have gone through similar things. That's why the charity myblackdog.co is such a wonderful idea. You get to talk to someone who has empathy because sympathy, as harsh as it sounds, isn't much help.

But apart from saying 'I'm not fine', what saved my life was the day I started doing the ironing ...

Act 3: The New Me

I lost count of the number of times Candy told me that one day I would get better. When you are lying in bed crying and you don't know why, that can be hard to believe. You will also find it impossible to believe you could emerge a stronger, better person. Yet you can.

Some people have to live with depression their whole life and can be constantly anxious and fearful that they will ruin every occasion from birthdays and weddings to Christmas. Sometimes just cleaning your teeth can feel well beyond you. And for many the drugs don't work.

Yet it turned out that the small breakthrough for me, with the value of hindsight, was when Candy suggested and I agreed to do one small activity each day that got me out of the bedroom and my dressing gown. That act was just to do ten minutes of ironing every day. I've no idea what might be the one small thing that could trigger a recovery in others but I'm willing to bet there is one.

However, the big breakthrough – when I began to feel a bit better – was when I realised how I had been abusing alcohol to get through the day and dampen my despair.

Trouble was it always returned once I sobered up.

In the past I had always associated drinking with having a good time and feeling good. But what happens if you start to drink *not* to be happy but to stop being miserable? What happens if you dislike yourself and the terrible thoughts you are having so much that you resort to anything to shut them up, to shut everything out, to close everything down and find the quickest way to oblivion. What happens if, to stop the daily mental torment, you start to use alcohol as a sedative, and lots of it? Where is that going to end?

Once I started feeling a bit better, I stopped drinking. At the time of writing this article that's over three years ago. Now, on the rare occasions when people ask me why I don't drink, I say: 'I discovered it's not good for my mental health.' If anyone ever pushes you to drink and you don't want to, maybe tell them the same thing. It shuts them up every time. You don't have to have been mentally unwell to say it. You just want to stay mentally fit. By the way, I could write a whole other chapter on how it's possible to be a fun-loving non-drinker and enjoy being in the pub but you wouldn't believe that either.

When I was unwell I'd lost my meaning and purpose, which had always been to help and inspire others. For a very long time I couldn't even help myself. When at last I did emerge from the darkness, it came back tenfold. That's why, for me at least, in the end it proved to be not just a lesson but a blessing. Indeed, in the depth of winter, I finally learned that there was in me an invincible summer.

Now for some more unbelievable showing off.

I think I'm now a far better version of my old self. The Duracell bunny has got his bounce back but with much more besides. I am grateful for and appreciate every precious day and spend far more time 'in the moment' than I ever did before. I discovered how much people really loved me and who my true friends were.

I also realised the intimate connection between mental and physical wellbeing. That's why, having stopped drinking at the age of 60, I joined my first ever gym at 61, took up running at 62, having done bugger-all exercise for over 35 years, and ran my first marathon just shy of 63. I even took up Pilates and yoga with a passion. I lost two stone but more importantly I gained not just physical but much more emotional strength and resilience. None of that would have happened if I'd not been ill.

Has the black dog totally disappeared? Very, very occasionally I hear him barking faintly in the distance but I now know what to do to stop him getting up close.

The best advice I can give you is if you suspect someone is mentally unwell ask them if they are OK. Even if they say 'I'm fine' I'd encourage you to ask them twice, especially if they are a man. This may just provide them with the courage to tell you how they truly feel. Maybe start by asking yourself twice.

Finally, if you are ill right now, I know you won't believe me when I tell you that at some time in the future, a future that I also know you cannot even begin to imagine, you will genuinely be fine and have become an even better version of your previous self. You may idly pick up this book again and think, 'If only I could have believed him back then!'

Until that big day comes, for now, just cling on to the small tiny things: the slight slivers of light that briefly shine in the darkness. You might start with a spot of ironing. And tell that black dog from me to f##k right off.

Afterword

From my wife Candy for those of you caring for someone who is depressed:

1. Always remember that the person you love is still there. The stranger that inhabits their body is the illness. They may act in a totally alien way. Depression is selfish, uncommunicative and isolating. Do not take this personally. None of this is your fault.

   And it is not your responsibility to fix it.

2. Fit your own oxygen mask first. It can be incredibly challenging to live with or love someone who is ill with depression. You have to take care of yourself first as a priority. It isn't being selfish, it's a necessity.

3. In particular it can be stressful dealing with all the people who know your loved one is ill and constantly ring or text for updates. They mean well but you may feel as though you are trying to support everyone around you as well as the person who is ill. Let them know you need their support, but it may be better for you to get in touch rather than the other way around.

4. Communicate. This is a tough one. It can be very, very difficult especially for men to talk about their feelings. In depression it's often impossible. Steve found that talking was far too hard at times. But

texting can help if the words don't come easily. Write a letter. Create a WhatsApp group of close friends, nearest and dearest, where the person who is ill can give them a score between 1 and 10 for how they are feeling today. They'll then know if they are up for a chat or a coffee.

5. Above all, do not get sucked into negativity. Remember it is an illness and that person can get better. Always, always have faith and hope.

About Steve

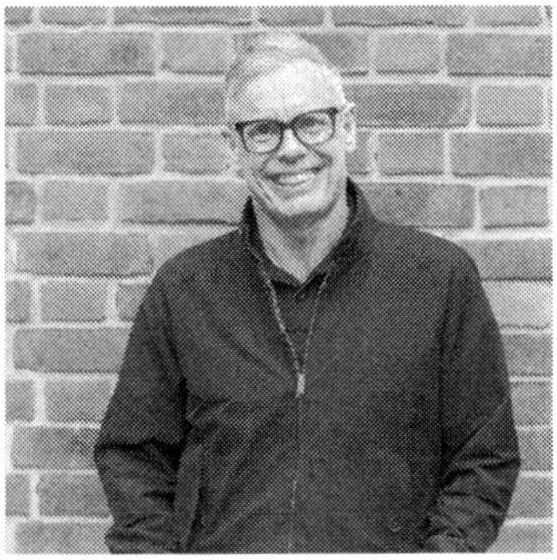

Steve McDermott has been speaking worldwide for over 25 years. (You'd have thought he would have run out of breath by now!)

He has won the European Motivational Speaker of the Year Award three times. The third edition of his International best-selling book "How to be a complete and utter f**k up: Forty-Seven and a half steps to lasting underachievement" is now available on Amazon.

Some describe him as the offspring between a stand-up comedian and self-improvement guru. He wouldn't.

When not speaking live and remotely at conferences and events, Steve's taught thousands of others the secrets of professional speakers through his company, the Confident Club.

He lives in Leeds with his wife Candy and Clive the rescue cat. That's Leeds, Yorkshire (in England), as no doubt Steve would be quick to point out.

Connect with Steve

www.linkedin.com/in/stevemcdermott

www.twitter.com/stevemcthinking

www.instagram.com/stevemcthinking/

www.stevemcdermott.com

www.confidentclub.com

To ask Steve to speak at your conference or company event either live or remotely email him at:

hello@stevemcdermott.com

Why 'The Other F Word'?

Jo Baldwin Trott

Editor

'Why are you, a woman, creating a book about men's health?' I've been asked this many times over the last six months. It's a really good question and my initial answer back then was different to the one I give now. Along with many of the authors in this book, I have been on a journey since I felt the need to create this book – one of my own acknowledgment and healing. Such is the power of acknowledging our experience and, as Maria Adriana Contreras explains, of leaving denial behind.

The journey of publishing my second book 'Silver Linings' (Proper Books, 2020), the positive stories of lockdown, was coming to an end when I received a message to create this book. I call them 'downloads' ... when you feel someone is with you even though the room is empty, and a voice from inside gives you a message. Shortly after, a very good friend in the wellbeing world who was in Silver

Linings asked me to create a book for men, a book to support men with their mental health.

A further two connections approached me and mentioned men's mental health and how little literature there was on the topic. Then, on my favourite radio station the DJ Eddy Temple-Morris spoke about being the patron of My Black Dog and how the demand for men's mental health support had gone through the roof since a virus spread across our planet.

And finally, I heard a shocking story from a fellow author in another book. Her husband had sadly passed on, and in the book she fully explained why and how. This was the final nudge I needed, and as Proper Books is focused on social consciousness, to help with a very current problem, it was an easy choice. But as a woman it's been a fascinating journey. I hope many women read this book because it is just as enlightening for women as it is for men.

Wearing a Mask

There are many conditions and traditional mindsets associated with being British; pretending and hiding our fears is just one of them. Author Raj Koria describes it as 'wearing a mask' and explains how he has only just realised, post-divorce, that he has been wearing a mask all of his life.

Sadly, it is a very normal state for a British person to hide what they're truly thinking and feeling. I have been surrounded by many men who have this mindset. I was brought up with this value of 'not making a fuss'. It didn't serve me well and I truly feel it is at the core of some of the depression and anxiety faced today. But wearing a mask is not just a British condition; it is a problem men face all over the world and Aboriginal man Jamie Marloo Thomas proves that in his words.

There are so many worries in our world right now that are new and previously never experienced. And these are on top of the normal concerns and pressures we have as parents, home-owners, renters, employees and employers. We have never needed to be more aware of what we say and the language we use. All these words count and land; each word has the potential to be heard or read by someone. These words deserve our attention, especially when they are coming from those we care about and those we hold dear.

As individuals, we need more than ever to be more honest with ourselves, especially when it comes to our mental health, and to encourage our loved ones to do the same. I am very concerned about our children's mental health post-virus and the ongoing psychological impact of mask-wearing, keeping our distance and the regular messages in the media to 'stay safe and stay at home'. One day our nation and our economy will have recovered from these times but the damage done to our children, especially young children, may take longer to recover from.

'Doctor avoidance' by men is often joked about but no one is laughing now. There should be no more joking over this mindset and this short-sighted moment of pride or conditioning to 'soldier on'. When it comes to physical and mental health it is even more crucial that men share their struggles before it gets too bad. This is the aim of the words in this book, to prevent others reaching the depths of depression and thoughts of suicide.

The Damage of Fine-ness

Sadly, I have experienced hearing the devastating words that someone close to me has taken their life not just once but a number of times. The youngest, a male, was just 16. I have also experienced loss as a consequence of 'fine-ness'.

In 2007 I lost my father, suddenly. He was 'just fine with a bit of heartburn' when he flew back to his home in West Africa in March 2007, but I never saw him again. He spent his last hours in a Gambian hospital still suffering with 'heartburn' – as the doctor had diagnosed – and was alone when his heart suddenly and fatally failed.

I was trained well in putting on a front and pretending all was well when it wasn't. I naturally attracted partners who were good at this, too.

The worst time of my life was shortly after my twin girls were born. They were tiny, three and a half months early and in intensive care when I drove to a car park and had that awful thought process of how, where, with what.

My marriage was struggling before the girls were born and now it was being tested to the limits.Thankfully, I eventually turned to my friends, or my 'soul sisters' as I call them. They were there for me, instantly, and listened. They supported me and didn't judge or 'there-there' me or problem-solve. They didn't try to fix anything. They just validated my struggles and sympathised, which was all I needed to help me get through another day, until eventually the days got easier and my babies' health got stronger. And eventually, I left my partner.

In my previous profession as a police officer I dealt with many desperate souls. Working in the most beautiful part of Bristol had its pluses but sadly its minuses too. The iconic Clifton Suspension Bridge attracted many people who were ready to end their lives. Three definitely didn't, not that day. But each desperate person had one thing in common: they felt alone and believed they had no one to share their fears with. And they were mostly men.

Gender and Vulnerability

I truly believe that women are generally 'allowed' and encouraged to open up more and consequently find it much easier to reach out to their friends and share their fears. Most women haven't had the training men have had – to 'man up', 'put a brave face on' and say, 'I'm fine'. Women generally have more friends and friends they are used to sharing their inner thoughts and worries with. We're used to being vulnerable. Generally, men are not and that needs to change.

Many of the authors in this book are creating opportunities within groups and safe spaces for men to speak openly and to share. As Mark Pitcher puts it, it is time to be brave and 'put down your proverbial shield'. It is time to be vulnerable and show other men how to be vulnerable, to show that it is okay and actually a fundamental part of being human.

Sharing our vulnerability and giving compassion are desperately needed now. Particularly now, men must know they can speak up, whether that is online to charities like My Black Dog or in men's support groups like those created by authors Kapil Gupta and Simon Walker, or to me or to you.

I am incredibly appreciative of every author in this book. They have shown vulnerability by sharing their experience to help you or someone you know. Some of the authors are sharing their story for the very first time, which is incredibly brave. They have all, however, recognised the importance of opening up, especially now. I am also grateful to the two female authors. I hope this book helps men everywhere to feel that women are supporting you; we are desperate to help.

I would like to give a very big thank you to Niki Clarke and the My Black Dog charity who are supporting our book. This groundbreaking charity recognises men like author Steve McDermott, who have struggled to say how bad they feel, and say these words out loud. My Black Dog offers peer-to-peer online support for you if you are struggling. Simply type in the words and share how you feel – you don't need to say them out loud.

Tragically the final nudge for me to create this book came from a fellow author from a previous book. She is Indian and was married to a man whom she described as 'typically British'. When he became ill with the coronavirus, instead of admitting how unwell he was, he insisted he was 'fine'. In fact, he kept repeating those words – until he wasn't, and was rushed into hospital. Sadly, it was too late. He has left his son father-less and his wife a widow.

Being honest rather than 'being fine' could save your life.

And if you hear the other 'f' word from a friend, a loved one, or even a stranger then ask them another question: 'Are you sure?' Ask them 'How are you really feeling?' or even 'What does fine mean to you?' It could save their lives.

Join our Being FINE weekly conversations live on Facebook in the *'Being FINE' Book. The other F word* group or via Proper Books Publishing on YouTube at:

www.youtube.com/channel/UCsxXtp1ecN8dSJ6upIJEwbw

Please go to www.myblackdog.co right now or contact the Samaritans www.samaritans.org (tel. 116123 UK/ email jo@samaritans.org and they will respond within 24 hours). You are not alone.

About Jo

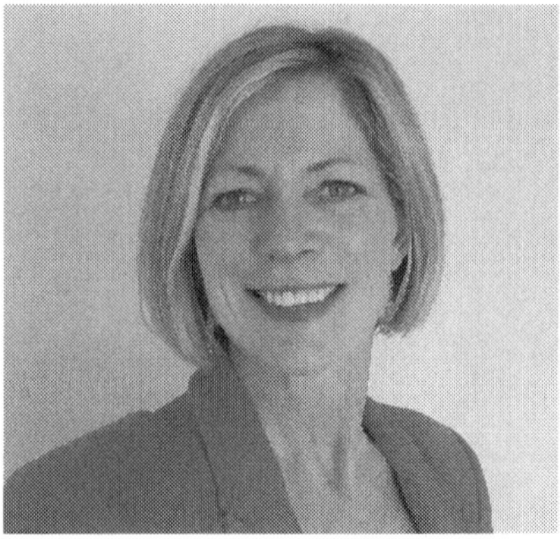

Jo Baldwin Trott is a leadership mentor and expert in personal brand.

She is an international bestselling author of *Women Leading* (Baldwin-Trott et al, 2020), *Fit for Purpose Leadership 6 & Remote Working* (Priestley et al, 2020) and her uplifting stories of lockdown, *Silver Linings,* is available on audio, Kindle and paperback.

As the founder and CEO of Proper Books Publishing, Jo creates books on social consciousness, addressing the issues of today.

Jo is a lecturer and professional speaker in business, personal brand and purpose.

Host of The Amijo Show, The Women Leading Show, Jo is also the founder of equality movement Women Leading

Global and director for the UK parliamentary equality group 5050 Parliament.

She is based in Hove, UK with her two children. She likes to write songs and be in the front row at live music events.

Join Jo's conversation on LinkedIn and all media via @jobaldwintrott.

Connect with Jo

www.jobaldwintrott.com

ProperBooksPublishing@gmail.com

Buy More of Jo's Proper Books

www.amazon.co.uk/Jo-Baldwin-Trott/e/B086MYX5NY

Printed in Great Britain
by Amazon

64325368R00099